KT-103-258

Massage Therapy Research

Tiffany Field PhD

Professor and Director, Touch Research Institutes, University of Miami School of Medicine, Florida, USA

Foreword by

Leon Chaitow ND DO

Registered Osteopathic Practitioner and Senior Lecturer, University of Westminster, London, UK; Editor, Journal of Bodywork & Movement Therapies

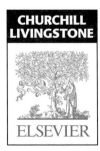

Edinburgh   London   New York   Oxford   Philadelphia   St Louis   Sydney   Toronto   2006

CHURCHILL LIVINGSTONE
ELSEVIER

An imprint of Elsevier Limited

First edition 2006

ISBN-10; 0443 102015
ISBN-13; 978-0-443-10138-0

British Library Cataloguing in Publication Data
A catalogue record for this book is available from the British Library.

Library of Congress Cataloging in Publication Data
A catalog record for this book is available from the Library of Congress.

Note
Neither the Publisher nor the Author assumes any responsibility for any loss or injury and/or damage to persons or property arising out of or related to any use of the material contained in this book. It is the responsibility of the treating practitioner, relying on independent expertise and knowledge of the patient, to determine the best treatment and method of application for the patient.

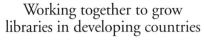

Printed in China

Contents

Foreword

Massage works. Massage eases pain—even in intractable settings. It also reduces psychological distress; modulates the effects of stress; improves sleep, mood and behavior; enhances circulation; encourages improved bowel and breathing function; and raises immunity—among many other benefits. The evidence is now so overwhelming as to the efficacy of massage therapy in these and a host of other diverse settings—from pregnancy to prematurity (and reducing the chances of prematurity), ADHD to autism, stroke to surgery, leukaemia to low back pain—that it is a wonder that government agencies, insurance companies and corporations are not falling over themselves to take advantage of this low-tech, safe, almost universally beneficial therapeutic approach!

Much of the credit for the research evidence is due to the untiring efforts of Tiffany Field and her team at the Touch Research Institutes (TRI), Miami School of Medicine. This new book is structured to lead the reader through the evolution of the benefits of massage therapy, from cradle to old age, from dysfunction to serious illness, as well as containing the bonus of a packed 80-page appendix that covers everything from A (aggression) to Y (yoga). This offers an extremely useful package of massage therapy abstracts, under 90 different headings. Many of the studies in this section derive from the Touch Research Institute, but by no means all do, emphasizing the growing interest of researchers world-wide.

Valuable information in the opening chapter describes the methods that have evolved at the TRI to meet the very special needs of research into massage therapy—from the formulation of a research question, through the processes of participant selection, procedures, protocols and finally to the analyses of statistics. In this age of evidence-based medicine this book should be essential reading for researchers into physical medicine, as well as practitioners and therapists within and outside those professions involved in bodywork and movement therapy.

In particular it should be read by health care professionals who are not yet aware of the value of massage—as well as by administrators and legislators associated with funding health care.

Leon Chaitow, 2005

Preface

Massage therapy existed before recorded time but only recently have research data documented its therapeutic effects. Positive outcomes include growth and development in preterm and full-term infants, as well as the treatment of attention deficits like autism and attention deficit hyperactivity disorder (ADHD); affective disturbances including depression, eating disorders and addictions; pain syndromes such as lower back pain and fibromyalgia; muscular problems from cerebral palsy to Parkinson's disease; autoimmune conditions like asthma and diabetes; and immune disorders such as HIV, leukemia and breast cancer. This book is a review of research studies from our laboratory on these conditions. These studies, as well as those from other laboratories that appear in the appendix abstracts, will hopefully help massage therapists and their students and clients to appreciate the benefits of massage, and help them understand the process by which we research those benefits.

Acknowledgements

I would like to acknowledge the people who have helped me conduct research on massage therapy, including my co-researchers, students, massage therapists and the participants in the research. This research was funded by grants from the National Institutes of Health, Department of Defense, March of Dimes, Biotone, Colgate–Palmolive and Johnson and Johnson Pediatric Institute.

Chapter 1

Massage therapy research methods

HISTORY OF MASSAGE THERAPY RESEARCH

Hippocrates said in 400 B.C. that 'medicine is the art of rubbing', a practice that came to be called massage therapy (Fig. 1.1). Published research on massage therapy dates back to the 1930s when human and animal studies were fairly popular. Several of those studies focused on documenting increased blood flow and reduced muscle atrophy associated with massage therapy. Although many of the research questions have remained the same over the years, the measurement technology has improved significantly. Early studies typically featured either single cases or very small samples. The samples were often self-selected clinical patients undergoing treatment for one or another condition. Measurement technology was limited to physiological measures including heart rate, blood pressure and temperature. Improved

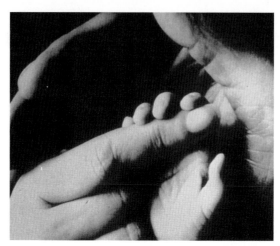

Figure 1.1 Touch.

technology for biochemical assays has enabled the testing of more expansive models and the exploration of underlying mechanisms.

The lack of control groups was another methodological problem. Without a control group, the effects of the massage could be due to 'placebo effects', the effects of simply receiving attention from a therapist. Control groups appeared in the literature more recently, but they were non-treatment control groups that could also benefit simply from attention by the therapist. More recently, massage therapy has been compared in studies to other therapies such as relaxation therapy. However, relaxation therapy requires work and concentration, so that the relaxation participants often did not complete the therapy sessions. To solve that problem, sham massage (light touch) groups are now being used as control groups.

FORMULATING THE RESEARCH QUESTION

The first question the readers should ask is whether the question addressed by the research is important and relevant to the field. The research question for most massage therapy studies is whether the therapy is effective and whether it is cost-effective for a particular condition. Interest in research often comes from personal interest, including family or friends having experienced a condition or because it is a common condition seen in therapists' practice, or simply, for the researcher, because the condition is a current funding priority and preliminary 'pilot' research is needed in order to obtain funding in that area. In order to show the effectiveness of the massage therapy the variables measured need to be meaningful. Meaningful variables are called 'gold-standard' variables or important clinical variables for that particular condition. It is then necessary to consider the most effective massage therapy technique for that condition. Also important is the selection of the most appropriate treatment comparison group and attention control group. To know whether and how these questions have been asked requires first a literature search, typically on the internet.

SEARCHING THE INTERNET FOR ALREADY EXISTING LITERATURE

Medline (www.medline.cos.com) and PsycINFO (www.apa.org/psycinfo) are the best-known literature search programs on the internet for current medical/psychological research, including massage therapy research. Literature from earlier decades can serve as a source of good ideas for replication studies using more sophisticated methods, but as, typically, current publications feature references from the last decade, literature searches are usually confined to the last decade. Another useful source that can be accessed by the general public is PubMed (provided by the National Center for Biotechnology Information) at www.ncbi.nlm.nih.gov.

The first step in conducting a literature search is to type the subject area (often referred to as a 'keyword') in the window that appears on the screen. A general topic of interest or a more specific area can be entered with the inclusion of the word 'and'. For instance, to find research on massage therapy, enter 'massage therapy'. However, if your interest is in researching the effects of massage therapy on a certain condition then you would enter 'massage therapy and fibromyalgia', for instance. This would enable you to access information on that particular area. In addition, if you are interested in research that includes massage therapy or fibromyalgia then entering 'massage therapy or fibromyalgia' would give you research articles involving either of those two areas. Once you have entered your particular subject of interest, a listing of citations that include that keyword will be shown. This citation includes the full reference for that research article, including author(s), title of article, journal in which it appears, volume number in which it can be found, page numbers, as well as the year it was published. Along with the reference an abstract is also provided. This is a brief summary of the research article that provides the most pertinent information of the study. If you decide to obtain the full article you now have all the necessary information in order to do so. Full articles for recent years are often available online. Older articles can be obtained from your local university library.

The literature search can be limited to the most current information available, or literature can be obtained from the last few decades. Terms for the condition along with the term massage therapy are likely to yield the most specific information needed. However, it is often good to start with a more global approach of entering the words 'treatment' or 'therapy' and the word for the condition. This general search would yield a greater number of abstracts and more general information about the condition; the hypothesized underlying etiology; gold-standard measures and other measures that have been used in research on other treatments of the condition; and ideas for treatment comparison groups that might serve as an attention control group. The material from the literature search then serves as the background or

introductory section or the first part of most published papers. Most researchers write the first half of the paper before starting the study in order to be
clear about the problem being addressed and the methods to study that
problem. The literature search can provide background on the incidence of
the problem; the symptoms; the etiology or potential etiology; previous treatments (both traditional and complementary); and the effectiveness of those
treatments. Once the background and methods sections are drafted, the paper
can serve as a proposal that can go to potential collaborators who could
facilitate the research.

SELECTING TREATMENT COMPARISONS AND ATTENTION CONTROL GROUPS

In most massage therapy studies over the years, the massage therapy subject
or group has been compared to a standard treatment control group, on assessments often made on the first and last days of the treatment period. The
problem with this comparison is that the participants might benefit from the
massage therapy simply because of the attention from the therapist. Thus,
researchers began to use treatment-comparison and/or attention control
groups. For example, in much of our early research we used relaxation therapy
as a comparison treatment group. Relaxation therapy had been shown to be
effective, especially in reducing stress and anxiety, mood states that typically
worsened the medical conditions we were studying. Another reason for using
relaxation therapy as a comparison group was to show that massage therapy
was more effective than relaxation therapy in order to justify the greater
expense of the massage therapy treatment. Unfortunately, relaxation therapy
was not an optimal treatment comparison group because the participants
found that relaxation therapy was hard work and required concentration and
self-discipline. Thus, the participants often 'skipped' their sessions and were
not compliant or cooperative with the treatment. In addition, relaxation was
often too difficult for young children because it required a certain amount of
cognitive sophistication along with a reasonable attention span. Thus, we
needed to use attention control conditions such as rocking the child, holding
the child and playing with toys, or holding and reading to the child.

More recently it was discovered that moderate pressure was necessary for
massage therapy to be effective (Diego et al 2004, Field et al 2004). Because
of that we have been using light pressure massage therapy as a comparison
group. The light pressure group receives exactly the same massage as the
moderate pressure group. This allows the subjects to be free of any expectations regarding results of their particular treatment. The participants in each
group would expect to receive some benefit from massage whether it was
deep pressure (in the case of the real treatment group) or light pressure (in
the case of the sham or placebo group). This also allows what is called 'double
blinding' or the possibility that the physicians who are providing the standard treatment and the massage therapists who are providing the massage
therapy do not necessarily have expectations that light or moderate pressure

massage is going to be more effective. In this way both the participants and the therapists are less biased about their treatment.

SELECTION OF PARTICIPANTS AND ASSIGNMENT TO GROUPS

Groups that are being compared need to be similar in terms of participants' characteristics, including age, gender, ethnicity and socioeconomic status or income. Generally, because all the participants are recruited at the same clinic (e.g. pediatric or adult clinic) and same facility, the age, ethnicity and socio-economic status are similar across participants. This helps prevent the group comparisons from being affected by variability of ethnicity or socioeconomic status. When participants are randomly assigned, like flipping a coin or drawing straws, the groups are expected to be roughly equivalent on these factors.

Severity of the medical condition is another critical background variable, particularly in medical research. Severity is often highly variable, suggesting the need for careful matching of groups. Participants are randomly assigned to groups by a table of random numbers, much like flipping a coin, or drawing straws, as already mentioned. Randomly assigning participants to groups is expected to yield roughly equivalent groups in terms of background variables. The most effective way to ensure similarity across groups is to match subjects across groups. For example, in studies on prematurely-born babies, the babies are frequently matched on birthweight and gestational age and then randomly assigned to treatment and control groups.

A less precise way is to use a random stratification procedure, assigning participants to different cells on a grid. For example, if there are two birthweight conditions (low birthweight and very low birthweight) and two gestational age conditions (short gestation and very short gestation), four cells would result (a cell for very short gestation and very low birthweight babies, a cell for very short gestation and low birthweight babies, a cell for short gestation and very low birthweight babies, and a cell for short gestation and low birthweight babies). A grid for these four cells would be prepared and subjects would then be randomly assigned to the 'cells' (the four groups) on this grid. Equal numbers of participants would be assigned to each of the four cells by the end of the study.

Determining the size of the sample involves several considerations. A power analysis is first conducted to determine what sample size is required to have enough statistical power for effects to be shown in the data analysis. Power can be determined by taking the difference between two group means (averages) from a previous study on a similar topic and dividing that difference by the larger of the two standard deviations for the same means. (The standard deviation reflects group variability.)

Even when the sample size is determined by a power analysis, other considerations such as economic constraints can keep the sample size to a minimum. One way to remain economical is by conducting data analyses as the group size is increased. For example, after recruiting 10 participants per group, data analyses can be conducted to determine whether the groups are significantly different on the key variables. If the groups are tending to differ statistically on those variables, then the absence of significant differences between groups may mean that the sample is too small and more participants need to be added. Researchers usually consider five participants per variable as a minimum sample for statistical analysis reasons.

SELECTING VARIABLES

The 'gold-standard' clinical variable, or the criterion for clinical improvement in any condition, is typically considered the most important variable. For example, in diabetes the 'gold-standard' variable is typically glucose level, and in asthma the 'gold-standard' variable is usually peak air flow. Clinical gold-standard measures are usually determined by collaborating physicians, based on already-existing research literature. Sometimes more than one clinical gold-standard measure is included.

Stress variables are a second important set of variables, because stress usually worsens clinical conditions. Self-report stress measures, such as the State Anxiety Index and the Profile of Mood State measures (to be elaborated later), are often used to assess stress. In addition, physiological measures, such as heart rate or blood pressure, and chemical measures, such as stress hormones (e.g. salivary cortisol), are good confirmatory measures for self-reported stress.

Treatment research usually involves assessment of the immediate effects of the therapy session, and the longer-term effects are assessed at the end of the treatment period. Follow-up assessments are sometimes conducted at 1 or 2 months after the end of the therapy period. The immediate effects of therapy can be measured by self-reports on the participant's anxiety level and mood state, and saliva samples are sometimes taken for a measure of stress hormone (the most common one being cortisol). Heart rate and blood pressure are common physiological measures of stress. Other measures are unique to the condition. For example, in the pain condition of juvenile rheumatoid arthritis, the response to a dolorimeter might be measured, the dolorimeter being a pressure gauge that determines the threshold beyond which the participant can no longer tolerate the pressure of the rod-like dolorimeter. In burn wound healing, the participant registers itching on a temperature gauge of itchiness immediately following the treatment. Longer-term measures are the gold standards or criteria for the effectiveness of the therapy. Those effects are indexed by clinical measures such as the number of back-pain-free days, number of migraine-free days, glucose levels, or pulmonary measures taken in children with asthma. Often clinical improvement is accompanied by decreases in depression and urinary stress hormones (e.g. cortisol and norepinephrine).

Sleep/wake behavior observations are also invaluable indicators of treatment and clinical changes. However, observers need to be trained to conduct live observations or to code videotapes of the behaviors if they have been videotaped, by checking off behaviors on paper grids, for example, every 10 seconds or on laptop computers second-by-second. Then at least two individuals need to observe and code behavior simultaneously to determine interobserver agreement (interobserver reliability). The standard for interobserver reliability is 90%, that is the two observers coded the behaviors similarly 90% of the total time sample units across usually one-third of the observations. Significant practice time is required to achieve this level of interobserver reliability. Interobserver reliability is calculated using a 'kappa coefficient', which is a statistical calculation that corrects disagreements that might happen by chance. Monitoring behavioral, physiological and biochemical measures simultaneously increases the robustness of the study. Self-report measures are usually taken on pencil and paper forms.

Heart rate and blood pressure are easily-recorded physiological assessments. More sophisticated measures such as vagal tone (derived from the respiratory sinus arrhythmia of heart rate) are more difficult to collect because of the technical equipment and labor-intensive data reduction required. Biochemical assays are rarely included in massage therapy studies because saliva and urine assays are expensive. For example, saliva cortisol assays cost approximately US$25.00 per sample. In most studies pre- and post-therapy saliva samples are taken on the first and last days of the study to total approximately US$100.00 per person.

Gold-standard clinical measures are typically performed by a physician, for example, pulmonary measures in children with asthma and the dolorimeter with patients with pain syndrome, such as those with fibromyalgia. Similar measures can sometimes be taken by the patient to corroborate the physician's assessment, for example, the peak air flow meter measuring pulmonary function by children with asthma and pain-rating scales by patients with fibromyalgia. When children are the participants in studies it is sometimes important to measure parental stress and mood state to determine whether the child's clinical course is affecting the parents and whether parental stress, in turn, may be affecting the child's clinical course.

THERAPY AND RESEARCH PROCEDURES

Treatment and research procedures need to be carefully considered and designed prior to the beginning of the study. Researchers write the background and the methods of their study in advance of their research so that the institution's review board can review any concerns they may have about protecting the rights of human subjects.

One of the most important aspects of the research procedure is that the participants and the observers should not know the hypotheses of the study and the participant's group assignment, as the participants and observers could be biased by these factors. Including several observers in the study can also help prevent bias, although the training of several observers and practice sessions to achieve interobserver reliability are costly.

The therapy protocol also requires careful thought. The description of the therapy needs to be extremely detailed to cover many muscle groups and different parts of the body to be effective. Cost considerations include the length of the session. This is relevant for both the cost of the study and the cost of transporting the treatment once it is determined to be effective. Most people cannot afford more than one 30-minute session by a professional massage therapist per week. Training a 'significant other' in the procedure is more cost-effective, although even that person is not likely to conduct massages more than a couple of times a week at 20–30 minutes per session. The research can be less expensive when using volunteer massage therapists. The therapists appreciate the research experience, particularly when it involves children, who they are rarely able to see otherwise. Participants are also more likely to continue their treatment if the procedure has proven cost-effective. For these reasons we have limited the therapy sessions in our studies to 20-minute sessions once or twice per week. We also train significant others to conduct the massage following the end of the study. They are given demonstrations on themselves and on the research participants and they are then given a video for home review of the procedure.

For massage studies with children, we teach the parents to be the therapists. The massage becomes part of the bedtime ritual that helps not only the children but the parents as well. We have documented that the therapist benefits from providing the massage in the same way that the recipient benefits (Field et al 1998a). Massage therapy by parents, of course, is a very cost-effective procedure and one that not only helps the child's clinical condition but also helps make the parent feel empowered as part of the treatment process and helps the parent's and child's relationship.

SELECTION OF COLLABORATORS

It is necessary for massage therapists wanting to conduct research to find research collaborators. Usually research collaborators can be found at universities or hospitals. The research protocol needs to be approved by an institutional review board in a research institution. Medical collaborators are important for identifying important clinical measures (gold standards) for the condition being studied. They can also refer patients for participation in research and can administer the clinical measures. Finally, they are helpful in terms of publications and grant proposals because they add credibility for reviewers of publications and grants. Scientist collaborators are also helpful. For example, neuroscientists can conduct assays of biochemical measures or interpret physiological data, e.g. electroencephalograms (EEGs). Statisticians and PhD researchers can assist with designing the methods and conducting the statistical analyses for the project. If the collaborating researcher is not a PhD-trained researcher, the team will need at least a statistician collaborator. Massage therapist collaborators are, of course, needed (particularly if the researcher is not a massage therapist), for the design of the massage therapy procedure to be used and to help identify measures that can directly assess the effects of that massage therapy procedure. Volunteer massage therapists are critical for the therapy itself or for demonstration of the therapy if the parents or significant others are going to be the therapists.

RESEARCH PROTOCOLS FOR SPECIFIC CONDITIONS

In the next section, specific research protocols are reviewed as examples. These include research on prenatal and postnatal growth and development, attention deficit hyperactivity disorder (ADHD), psychiatric conditions and addictions, pain syndromes, autoimmune conditions including asthma, dermatitis and diabetes, and immune conditions including HIV and breast cancer.

Growth and development studies

Pregnancy massage

Prematurity is a costly problem that would best be prevented. Stress and depression of the mother may contribute to prematurity. In some studies, for example, the cortisol levels (representative of stress) of the pregnant woman at 28 weeks' gestation predicted premature delivery with a reliability of 0.98 (Wadwha et al 1998). The prematurely-born babies had significantly higher cortisol levels than those who were not born prematurely. In another study conducted by our group, the mothers' prenatal catecholamines (norepinephrine) and stress hormones (cortisol) during the last trimester of gestation were later mimicked by their newborns (Lundy et al 1998). This finding concurs with data showing that at least 40% of the mother's cortisol crosses the placenta (Glover et al 1999). Another study from our laboratory suggests that fetuses of depressed versus non-depressed mothers were also more active from the fifth to the seventh gestational month (Dieter et al 2001), which may be a result of increased stress hormone levels. These data highlight the importance of interventions during pregnancy that can reduce stress and depression. In a recent study we provided pregnancy massage twice a week over the last trimester of pregnancy (Field et al 1998b). Perinatal complications were reduced, and most importantly, prematurity was reduced. In a more recent study we explored the effects of pregnancy massage specifically on depressed mothers (Field et al 2004). The massage reduced not only depression and anxiety but also the neurotransmitters and hormones associated with depression and anxiety (norepinephrine and cortisol). Serotonin, the antidepressant neurotransmitter, was increased. Again, reduced prematurity was the most important effect.

Labor massage

To continue the stress reduction achieved in pregnancy we taught significant others to perform labor massage (Field et al 1998b). In that study we were able to reduce labor pain by having the significant other give the massage for the first 15 minutes of every hour of labor. The massage led to shorter labors, less need for labor medication, shorter hospitalization and less postpartum depression.

Preterm growth and development

Approximately 10% of infants in the US are born prematurely at less than 37 weeks' gestation. Those infants are hospitalized in neonatal intensive care units (NICUs) for sometimes 2–5 months, experiencing stresses of the nursery including loud sounds and bright lights. When the newborn is no longer considered to be medically unstable, the primary agenda for the infant is to gain enough weight to be discharged. It is at this time that we have introduced 'preemie massage'. The massage protocol included three 15-minute massages a day for a 10-day period which led to a 47% greater weight gain (Field et al 1986). In our most recent study we were able to establish the same weight gain over a 5-day period (Dieter et al 2003) and thus we are now using the more cost-effective 5-day treatment period. We are also working to teach the parents to continue the massage following discharge.

In addition to weight gain, we documented that we could save US$4.7 billion in hospital costs if we were to provide 10 days of massage to the approximately 470 000 infants born prematurely in the US each year (saving US$10 000 in hospital costs per infant) due to their being discharged on average 6 days earlier. The cost savings would be even greater today because of increased NICU costs. We also observed sleep/wake behaviors and conducted newborn behavior assessments with these infants (see Appendix, p. 21 for the sleep/wake behavior codes and the list of behaviors). Recording 45-minute sleep/wake sessions, we were able to document that indeterminate sleep (a sleep state that is very difficult to code because it is disorganized and does not look like deep sleep or active sleep) was a problem for preterm infants, a problem that was diminished by the massage therapy. Also, the massaged babies were more responsive on the newborn assessments. Follow-up assessments showed that these infants still had a weight and developmental advantage at 8 months post-discharge (Scafidi et al 1993). Perhaps because their newborn behavior was more responsive, the infants' interactions with their parents were better and thus, they were able to eventually show better growth and development.

We later added growth hormone (IGF1) and oxytocin to our set of measures. These variables are considered important for growth and have been shown to increase with additional stimulation in rats, for example (Uvnas-Moberg 1993). We added these variables in order to explore the underlying mechanism for the massage therapy/weight-gain relationship. In an earlier study we speculated that the underlying mechanism for increased weight gain in the massaged preterm babies was that following massage the activity of the vagus nerve was increased. As a result more food absorption hormones were being released for more efficient food absorption, that being the function of the vegetative branch of the vagus nerve. Vagal activity was measured from heart rate recordings and was shown to increase, and insulin (a food absorption hormone) in plasma samples increased. Other possible underlying mechanisms include an increase in gastric motility (also stimulated by the vegetative branch of the vagus nerve), which could also contribute to more efficient food absorption.

The additional measures of IGF1 and oxytocin may further inform us as to underlying mechanisms. If underlying mechanisms are known, medical professionals are more likely to adopt massage therapy as a routine treatment on neonatal intensive care units. Functional magnetic resonance imaging (MRI) methods are being used by some researchers to show that significant brain development accompanies massage therapy, particularly the development of the hippocampus (the brain region that involves memory functions). In the rat, which often serves as a model for human growth and brain development, increased dendritic arborization (branching) occurs in the hippocampal region following moderate-pressure rubbing (Schanberg & Field 1987). In this study, the experimenter used a paintbrush to simulate the mother's moderate-pressure tongue licking. The tongue-licking pressure lowered levels of cortisol, which is noted to kill brain cells. Brain cells were saved, and as adults, the rats performed maze tests as well as they had in their youth.

Unfortunately, the use of functional MRI and growth measures (IGF1 and oxytocin) are extremely expensive in the human. For example, IGF1 growth hormone assays cannot be done until dozens of samples are collected because of the expense involved in assaying a few samples at a time. Functional MRI equipment and the technical expertise that is needed to read the functional MRI scans are extremely expensive. Although brain scans and growth hormones are compelling data, the clinical measure, in this case weight gain, is typically the easiest and least expensive variable.

Attention and attention disorders

Stimulation of the vagus is critical for attention. Vagal activity and EEG patterns are reliable indicators of attention; slower heart rate and increased vagal activity accompany attention. The sinus arrhythmia of heart rate is controlled by the vagus, so heart rate recordings can be easily converted to vagal activity by a computer program. EEG requires sophisticated equipment and technical expertise for reducing the data. EEG patterns that accompany attentiveness include increased beta and theta waves. This EEG pattern of heightened alertness/attentiveness was noted in a recent study following 15-minute chair massages in participants' offices (Field et al 1997a). The EEG alertness/attentiveness pattern following the massage sessions was accompanied by improved performance on mathematical computations, including being able to perform them in less time with greater accuracy. Enhanced performance has also been documented for infants (Cigales et al 1997). That study showed superior performance on habituation tasks by infants following massage. These are primitive learning tasks involving learning that a repeated stimulus, such as the repeated sound of a bell, becomes irrelevant because it does not signal anything else happening. The infant stops responding to the stimulus and then responds to a novel stimulus, suggesting that the old stimulus was learned. We also showed in a study on preschool children that they were able to perform IQ scale items including pegs and block design tasks in less time and more accurately following a brief massage (Hart et al 1998).

Children with attention disorders

Children with attention disorders such as autism (Field et al 1997b) and ADHD (Field et al 1998c) are also able to perform better and stay on task for longer periods following massage therapy. After two sessions per week by a massage therapist these children were able to stay on task longer and relate more to their teachers (Field et al 1997b). In a more recent study the children's parents were used as the therapists (Escalona et al 2001). That study showed that the children not only spent more time being attentive and on-task in the classroom, but they also showed fewer sleep problems. Sleep problems are prevalent in children with autism. The sleep diaries kept by the parents on the onset of sleep, duration of sleep and number of sleep-wakings were a critical measure. To the parents' surprise, sleep problems decreased over this brief period.

Parents of children with autism are often biased toward seeing any signs of improvement. Thus, converging measures are particularly important. In some studies we have recorded night-time sleep by time-lapse video. With time-lapse video 8 hours of sleep, for example, can be coded in 1 hour. The taped movements look like Charlie Chaplin moving about, so they are easy to record for a measure of activity. Activity is only seen in active sleep (versus deep sleep). Night-wakings and moving out of the bed are coded as wakeful activity. Actometers (activity monitors) are more precise measures of sleep, they are less intrusive and they require less subject compliance. The actometer is a converted Timex watch (with the spring removed) such that every time a participant moves an arm, the time hand on the watch moves. The clock time elapsed on the watch from night-time to daytime is a measure of activity that has occurred during night-time sleep. This becomes the total time in active sleep or non-deep sleep. Actometers are easy to use with all age groups.

Similar measures have been used with children and adolescents with ADHD (Field et al 1998c). The most meaningful measures for this group are those taken in the classroom, where the children show their worst problems. In studies on ADHD teacher and parent rating scales were used (the Conners scale because it is shorter than the Child Behavior Checklist, a similar measure used by parents and teachers). Parents' and teachers' ratings often correlate. Some behaviors are difficult for parents to rate, for example, on-task behavior in the classroom, and some are difficult for teachers to rate, for example, sleep behavior. Teachers' and parents' ratings have been criticized because they are thought to be subjective. However, they have recently been highly correlated with independent observer ratings, so they are now less subject to criticism.

Attentiveness would ideally be recorded by some kind of device that could be mounted on the head to record eye movements and free field recordings of heart rate that would not be affected by movement. However, when sophisticated devices are used, their readings are often similar to (correlated with) behavior ratings. For example, EEG sleep recordings are highly correlated with activity watch (actometer) readings of sleep activity as well as time-lapse video recordings of activity.

Psychiatric conditions

Psychiatric conditions such as depression or eating disorders and post-traumatic stress disorder (PTSD) can also be improved by massage therapy. Because these are typically accompanied by depressed mood and anxiety, we include self-reports on depression and anxiety in our studies. These include:

1. The Profile of Mood States (McNair et al 1971), which taps depressed mood state, anxiety, and anger.
2. The Center for Epidemiological Studies on Depression Scale (CESD; Radloff 1977) or the Beck Depression Inventory (Beck et al 1961), both of which measure depressive symptoms. The CESD seems to be more sensitive (detects more individuals with depressive symptoms) and is more user-friendly or simpler. Younger and less educated people are more able to complete this instrument.
3. The State Anxiety Inventory (Spielberger et al 1970) (which also has a children's version called the State Anxiety Inventory for Children [STAIC]), assesses state anxiety (current, short-term anxiety) and trait anxiety (approximating a personality trait). The State–Trait Anger Expression Inventory (STAXI), designed by the same psychologist, measures anger. These 20-item, five-point scales are easy to complete and have good properties including good test–retest reliability (meaning that completing the scale on two occasions usually yields similar ratings).

For an assessment of psychiatric conditions we also use converging measures of behavior including the symptoms that are reported on the self-report scales, for example, depressed affect, anxious and angry behavior. For behavior observations we designed the Behavior Observation Scale. Following a brief behavior observation the behaviors are rated on a five-point scale. Both mood scales are completed by the participant, and the behavior observations are made before and after the massage therapy session.

A third set of measures typically collected for individuals with psychiatric conditions are saliva (for an assay of the stress hormone cortisol) before and after the first and last massage therapy session. Urine is collected for assays of the stress neurotransmitters (norepinephrine and epinephrine), the body's natural antidepressants (dopamine, serotonin), and cortisol, at the beginning of the first and last sessions of the treatment period. The saliva measure of cortisol is taken as an index of the immediate reduction of stress following the therapy session, and the urine assays are made to assess the longer-term effects of massage therapy over the course of the study.

The above, self-help, behavior observations, and biochemical samples have been included in our studies on depressed children, depressed adolescents and depressed mothers, as well as studies conducted on patients with eating disorders (anorexia, bulimia) to assess the longer-term effects of massage therapy. Depression, eating disorders and addictions are considered to have an underlying depression base. This suggests the use of depression measures across studies. Other measures that were unique to the different studies included:

1. Time-lapse videotaped sleep during a child and adolescent psychiatry study as well as nurses' ratings of the children's and adolescents' behavior on the the psychiatric unit.
2. The Eating Disorders Inventory (Garner et al 1983) for an eating disorder study.
3. The number of cravings and cigarettes smoked for a smoking cessation study.
4. EEG for depressed adult studies. Relative right frontal EEG is typically noted in depressed individuals during the expression or reception of negative emotions. The right frontal area of the brain is involved in processing negative emotions. Less right frontal EEG activation is noted following massage therapy.
5. For children with PTSD (following Hurricane Andrew), the children drew themselves using magic markers to assess the change in depression. The drawings are scored on seven factors including: (1) small figure on page; (2) use of dark colors; (3) missing facial features; (4) sad face; (5) distorted figure; (6) displaced body parts; and (7) agitated lines. The drawings of depressed children often have very few facial features, distorted body parts and a small figure on the page.

Pain syndromes

A number of pain syndromes have shown benefit from massage therapy, including migraine headaches, lower back pain, premenstrual syndrome, and pain from burns, fibromyalgia and juvenile rheumatoid arthritis. In these conditions we have used self-report scales on pain including the McGill pain questionnaire, the pain intensity scale and a visual analog scale such as a ruler with ratings along its scale or a thermometer with ratings in the case of adults or a series of sad to happy faces in the case of children's ratings of pain. In addition to children's selection of faces that match their feelings, we often ask the children's parents and physician to rate the pain they think the child is experiencing. We also use measures unique to the different syndromes. So, for example, for migraine headaches, participants are asked to keep a diary on their headache-free days.

For lower back pain we assessed range of motion and the patients' ability to touch their toes. For burn subjects higher pain thresholds were noted following the massage therapy sessions. Their reactions to debridement (skin brushing) were assessed to determine their pain threshold. For fibromyalgia we used a dolorimeter (a rod that exerts pressure until the patient winces, representing the pain threshold). For juvenile rheumatoid arthritis, we asked parents to assess their child's ability to continue activities of daily living.

Because pain syndromes are often accompanied by anxiety, and anxiety in turn exacerbates pain syndromes, we also use anxiety scales (State Anxiety Inventory) to assess the pre- and post- massage therapy session anxiety levels. In addition, we use saliva cortisol as a secondary measure of anxiety/stress levels pre- and post-massage therapy sessions. Sleep is disturbed in pain syndromes either because of the pain or because sleep disturbances contribute to the pain (the direction of this relationship is not certain). Thus, we have used sleep recordings (sleep diaries or actometers). More recently we have noticed that sleep improved following massage therapy in pain syndromes, and pain was also reduced. Pain syndromes are often accompanied by insufficient deep or restorative sleep. Reduced deep sleep is accompanied by increased levels of substance P which causes pain. In a recent study on fibromyalgia we noted reduced substance P in saliva samples, improved sleep and decreased pain following a 1-month massage therapy treatment period.

Autoimmune disorders

Stress hormones such as cortisol are known to interact with and to affect autoimmune and immune conditions. Thus, cortisol is measured in saliva before and after massage therapy sessions and in urine at the beginning and end of the study period. In autoimmune diseases in children (including asthma, dermatitis, and diabetes), parents were used as the massage therapists. We knew that the parents would also likely benefit from the therapy because we had noted improvement in elderly volunteer massage therapists who massaged infants. The volunteers became less depressed, and their cortisol levels decreased (Field et al 1998a). We also know that parents' stress levels affect their children's stress levels, which may in turn affect their autoimmune condition. Thus, we also use self-report measures to assess stress in parents. The other measures of the autoimmune conditions are unique to the condition.

In the case of diabetes, self-report measures are completed by the parents on the child's glucose regulation, insulin and food regulation and exercise. In addition, glucose levels are measured by the children and their parents using a calibrated glucometer. The readings are taken at the same time of day by the parents. Measures such as fructosamine and glycosylated hemoglobin help confirm the diabetes condition.

The 'gold-standard' measures in dermatitis (eczema) following massage therapy included the following in both the focal area and the global area of the dermatitis:

- redness
- lichenification (thickening and hardening of the skin, often resulting from the irritation caused by repeated scratching)
- scaling
- excoriation (an abrasion typically from scratching)
- pruritus (the symptom of itching).

These were rated on a scale of 0–3 by a dermatologist and a dermatology fellow, who were unaware of the child's group assignment.

The gold-standard clinical measure for asthma is the peak air flow meter value recorded by children or their parents. Typically these are done on a daily basis, and the recorded value is entered into a diary. A pulmonologist also monitored at least four standard pulmonary measures at the beginning and the end of the study, including forced vital flow capacity, forced expiratory volume, average flow rate, and peak expiratory flow.

Immune disorders

Natural killer cells and natural killer cell activity were invariably increased after massage therapy in all of our immune studies including HIV in adults (Ironson et al 1996), HIV in adolescents (Diego et al 2001), and breast cancer (Hernandez-Reif et al 2003). Natural killer cells are considered the front line of the immune system, and they ward off viral and cancer cells. A recent theory suggests that they may even be substitutes for the destroyed CD4 cells in HIV. Thus, we invariably assay natural killer cell number and natural killer cell activity (see Appendix 2 for the immune measures typically assayed). In the study on men with HIV, the immune systems of the men were so compromised, and their CD4 cell numbers (the cells killed by HIV) were so low that it was not possible to reverse those numbers. In the less immune-compromised HIV adolescents of our more recent study, we were able not only to increase natural killer cells, but also to increase the CD4 cell numbers. Like the other conditions we have studied, these immune conditions are highly affected by stress hormones. Stress hormones such as cortisol kill immune cells. Thus, we have also assayed cortisol levels.

STATISTICAL ANALYSES

Statisticians and PhD-level researchers are trained in statistical analysis. Although using statistical analysis software is like following a recipe, knowing the appropriate statistics to use and how to interpret the results is the work of an expert in this area. The basics are briefly described below.

In any comparison of treatment groups, the scores or values of the variables are added and the total is divided by the number of participants to obtain the mean/average score, rating or value. The distance of individuals' scores from the mean is called variability or variance. Variance is typically indicated by standard deviations, with three standard deviations above the mean and three below the mean covering the distribution. A typical distribution of scores would have a mean in the middle of a line with most of the individuals falling near the mean, but as individuals' scores differ from the mean, they are farther out on the line either to the left or to the right of the center. To give an example, the mean IQ score for the population at large is 100. However, many individuals receive higher scores and many receive lower scores on this normal IQ distribution. One standard deviation from the mean is 16 points higher or a score of 116 (which would be considered above average), or 16 points lower or a score of 84 (which would be considered below average). Two standard deviations would be 2×16 or 132 (which would be considered gifted) or 68 (which would be considered retarded). Very few people would be out beyond two standard deviations. Standard deviation is the term for variability.

For group comparisons, the t-test is one of the simplest statistics performed. Group means and standard deviations are entered into an equation to calculate a t-value. The t-value is then considered statistically significant if this value could happen only five times out of a hundred or significantly more often than chance (which would be 5 in 100 times) (described as 'at $p \leq 0.05$ level' in a publication). Typically, t-values greater than 2.00 are significant. The t-test can be performed by hand on a calculator or using a software program such as SPSS, BMDP, or SAS on the computer. A printout provides the significance levels, or t-values can be found in a table of t-values in a statistics textbook and the p level or significance level checked in that table. The significance level only indicates whether the test result was statistically significant, suggesting that the groups compared were significantly different on that score or value.

Another statistical test for group comparisons is called the F test. The F test is basically the same as a t-test but is performed when more than two groups are being compared or when two groups are being compared at two different times. The analysis of variance (ANOVA) is the statistical test used to calculate an F value. An F test can also be found on the computer printout or checked in a statistics book table to determine the p level. Typically, F values greater than 4.00 are significant.

When more than two groups are being compared on more than three variables, more complex ANOVAs called MANOVAs (multivariate analyses of variance) can be performed. A MANOVA is performed on the group of variables for all groups to determine whether the groups generally differ on the group of variables. If the MANOVA F is significant, then post-hoc ANOVAs are conducted on each of the variables. The MANOVA F is again checked for a p level, which indicates whether the groups are significantly different on the group of variables as a whole. Subsequently, the F values from the individual variable ANOVAs and their p levels indicate whether the groups are different on each of the individual variables.

If there is more than one independent variable describing the group, for example, age and gender, the MANOVAs and ANOVAs could yield significant group differences on age and gender. They could also yield age by gender interaction effects meaning that one particular age of one particular gender differs from the other possible combinations. For example, young females could outperform young males, older females and older males on speed of reflexes. To test this interaction effect it would be necessary to conduct post-hoc t-tests to test all the possible comparisons including young females versus old females versus young males versus old males.

Variables can also be related to each other, and the data can be examined for the relationships between the variables. For example, anxiety scores may be related to gender such that higher anxiety scores are noted for males versus females. A correlation analysis (analysis of relationships between variables) can be conducted on the entire group of variables. The computer program prints a matrix of correlation coefficients that range from 0 (no relationship) to 0.99 (a perfect relationship). If the correlation between gender and anxiety is 0.83, those variables are highly correlated or strongly related. If anxiety scores run from low to high with higher values reflecting higher anxiety and males are classified as a 2 (and females as a 1), the relationship between gender and anxiety is 0.83 or a positive relationship suggesting males are more anxious. If males were more anxious but had been assigned a value of one, the correlation would be a −0.83 or a negative (or inverse) relationship. Again, the table of numbers is checked for the p level (if the computer output does not provide a p level).

More complex analyses on the relationships between variables can be conducted. For example, stepwise regression analyses can determine the relative importance of the predictor variables or the independent variables (the variables that affect an outcome). Again, if we are talking about age, gender and anxiety we could enter into the stepwise regression analysis the anxiety scores as the dependent measure (or the outcome variable), and gender and age would be entered as the predictor variables. If gender is highly correlated with anxiety (0.83), as was already noted, gender would be entered as a potential predictor variable into the equation. This statistical result in a stepwise regression would be interpreted as explaining 64% of the outcome variance. The variance (or R^2) can be obtained by multiplying the correlation coefficient (r) by itself ($0.83 \times 0.83 = 0.64$). This would tell you how much the variable gender is contributing to the outcome anxiety variable (64%). If age was entered into the equation at the second step or was the second most important predictor variable and the correlation coefficient was 0.91 with an R square of 0.81 or 81% ($0.91 \times 0.91 = 0.81$) the age variable group comparison would have added 17% to the variance (64% + 17% = 81%). Again, p levels would be given to indicate statistical significance.

These are some of the simplest statistical analyses performed in treatment group comparison research. Sometimes they cannot be used because, for example, the data are not normally distributed or they are 'skewed'. Then the use of non-parametric statistics (instead of the parametric statistics just described) would be indicated. The database needs to meet the required assumptions, for example, that the data be normally distributed in order to perform parametric analyses. These considerations are complex, and understanding statistical analyses as well as using them appropriately and not overinterpreting or overgeneralizing from the results requires considerable expertise in statistics.

SUMMARY

Therapists can learn basic statistics to understand and be able to critically evaluate the research reports they read. But to conduct research it is necessary to collaborate with trained researchers to design the study, including the treatments and measures, to obtain institution review board permission to conduct the study, to monitor quality of the data collection and computer entry, and to conduct and interpret data analyses. This collaboration between therapists and scientists throughout the scientific process is critical for improving and advancing the research methodology and for addressing the important questions in the field.

Summaries of our studies are presented throughout this book to give you a more detailed description of how we conduct research. In Appendix 2, abstracts are presented from quality massage therapy research studies in the literature. They are included to inform you of the most recent massage therapy research findings on a variety of conditions and to inform your clients. As you will note, the findings are invariably positive. This phenomenon could relate to negative findings rarely being published and to the more likely possibility that massage therapy is an effective treatment for many reasons for many conditions.

References

Beck A, Ward C, Mendelson M, et al 1961 An inventory for measuring depression. Archives of General Psychiatry 4:561–571.

Cigales M, Field T, Lundy B, et al 1997 Massage enhances recovery from habituation in normal infants. Infant Behavior and Development 20:29–34.

Diego MA, Hernandez-Reif M, Field T, et al 2001 HIV adolescents show improved immune function following massage therapy. International Journal of Neuroscience 106:35–45.

Diego MA, Field T, Sanders C, et al 2004 Massage therapy of moderate and light pressure and vibrator effects on EEG and heart rate. International Journal of Neuroscience 114:31–44.

Dieter J, Field T, Hernandez-Reif M, et al 2001 Maternal depression and increased fetal activity. Journal of Obstetrics and Gynaecology 21:468–473.

Dieter JN, Field T, Hernandez-Reif M, et al 2003 Stable preterm infants gain more weight and sleep less following 5 days of massage therapy. Journal of Pediatric Psychology 28(6):403–411.

Escalona A, Field T, Singer-Strunk R, et al 2001 Brief report: improvements in the behavior of children with autism following massage therapy. Journal of Autism and Developmental Disorders 31:513–516.

Field T, Schanberg SM, Scafidi F, et al 1986 Tactile/kinesthetic stimulation effects on preterm neonates. Pediatrics 77:654–658.

Field T, Quintino O, Henteleff T, et al 1997a Job stress reduction therapies. Alternative Therapies 3:54–56.

Field T, Lasko D, Mundy P, et al 1997b Brief report: autistic children's attentiveness and responsivity improved after touch therapy. Journal of Autism & Developmental Disorders 27(3):333–338.

Field T, Hernandez-Reif M, Quintino O, et al 1998a Elder retired volunteers benefit from giving massage therapy to infants. Journal of Applied Gerontology 17:229–239.

Field T, Hernandez-Reif M, Taylor S, et al 1998b Labor pain is reduced by massage therapy. Journal of Psychosomatic Obstetrics and Gynecology 18:286–291.

Field T, Quintino O, Hernandez-Reif M, et al 1998c Adolescents with attention deficit hyperactivity disorder benefit from massage therapy. Adolescence 33:103–108.

Field T, Hernandez-Reif M, Diego M, et al 2004 Massage therapy by parents improves early growth and development. Infant Behavior and Development 27:435–442.

Garner DM, Olmstead MP, Polivy J 1983 The Eating Disorders Inventory: a measure of cognitive behavioral dimensions of anorexia nervosa and bulimia. In: Darby PL, Garfinkel PR, Garner DM, et al (eds) Anorexia nervosa: recent development in research. Alan R Liss, New York, p 173–184.

Glover V, Teixeira J, Gitau R, et al 1999 Mechanisms by which maternal mood in pregnancy may affect the fetus. Contemporary Reviews in Obstetrics and Gynecology 24:1–6.

Hart S, Field T, Hernandez-Reif M, et al 1998 Preschoolers' cognitive performance improves following massage. Early Child Development & Care 143:59–64.

Hernandez-Reif M, Ironson G, Field T, et al 2003 Breast cancer patients have improved immune and neuroendocrine functions following massage therapy. Journal of Psychosomatic Research 1:1–8.

Ironson G, Field T, Scafidi F, et al 1996 Massage therapy is associated with enhancement of the immune system's cytotoxic capacity. International Journal of Neuroscience 84:205–218.

Lundy B, Jones NA, Field T, et al 1998 Prenatal depressive symptoms and neonatal outcome. Infant Behavior and Development 22:121–137.

McNair DM, Lorr M, Droppleman LF 1971 POMS—Profile of Mood States. Educational and Industrial Testing Services, San Diego, CA.

Radloff L 1977 The CES-D scale: a self-report depression scale for research in the general population. Applied Psychological Measures 1:385–401.

Scafidi F, Field T, Schanberg SM 1993 Factors that predict which preterm infants benefit most from massage therapy. Journal of Developmental and Behavioral Pediatrics 14(3):176–180.

Schanberg S, Field T 1987 Sensory deprivation stress and supplemental stimulation in the rat pup and preterm human neonate. Child Development 58:1431–1447.

Spielberger CD, Gorusch TC, Lushene RE 1970 The State Trait Anxiety Inventory. Consulting Psychologists Press, Palo Alto, CA.

Uvnas-Moberg K 1993 Role of efferent and afferent vagal nerve activity during reproduction: integrating function of oxytocin on metabolism and behavior. Psychoneuroendocrinology 19:687–695.

Wadwha PD, Porto M, Garite TJ, et al 1998 Maternal corticotropin releasing hormone levels in the early third trimester predict length of gestation in human pregnancy. American Journal of Obstetrics and Gynecology 179:1079–1085.

APPENDIX

Sleep states and Brazelton Neonatal Behavior Assessment Scale

Sleep states
Deep
Light
Drowsy
Alert
Active
Crying
Brazelton items
In sleep
  Flashlight
  Rattle
  Bell
Uncover
Pin prick
Ankle clonus
Foot grasp (plantar)
Babinski
Undress
Passive movements arms___legs___
General tone
Hold
Palmar grasp____ pull-to-sit _____
Standing ____ walking ____
Placing ____ incurvation ____
Body tone ____ crawling ____
Rooting _____ sucking ____
Nystagmus ____ glabella _____
Cuddliness ____ tonic deviation ____
Orientation
Inanimate visual (ball)
Inanimate auditory (rattle)
Inanimate auditory and visual (rattle)
Animate visual (face)
Animate auditory (voice)

Brazelton behaviors
State changes
  Predominant states
  Number of changes
Self quieting
Attempts
Brief (5 seconds)
Successful (15 seconds)
Hand to mouth
None
Swipes
Contact
Insertion
Startles
Tremulousness
Skin color
Irritable crying
Pull-to-sit
Uncover
Pin prick
Undress
Tonic neck reflex
Prone
Moro reflex
Defensive

Animate auditory and visual
Return to bassinette
Defensive (cloth on face)
Tonic neck reflex
Moro reflex

Chapter **2**

Reducing prematurity

The current rate of prematurity in the US is approximately 13%. Although the causes of prematurity are not yet known, elevated stress hormones (cortisol and corticotropic-releasing hormone) are noted to predict prematurity (Wadhwa et al 1998). Massage therapy has been noted to reduce cortisol levels in several studies (Field et al 1999, 2004), and massage therapy during pregnancy has been noted to reduce the prematurity rate in the same studies. In the first study in this chapter, pregnant women were noted to benefit from massage therapy not only by reducing their own leg and back pain but also by reducing obstetric complications, especially the prematurity rate (Field et al 1999). In the second study, a more cost-effective massage therapy was delivered by the woman's significant other (Field et al 2004). In this study, the prematurity rate was also reduced. In the third study we began to explore the effects of massage stimulation on fetal activity (Diego et al 2002). In that study a comparison was made between massaging a mother's feet and hands. Early in pregnancy there was seemingly only a response to the foot massage.

STUDY 1: PREGNANT WOMEN BENEFIT FROM MASSAGE THERAPY

Back and leg pain during pregnancy may lead to difficulty sleeping due to discomfort and body pains (Heliovaara 1989). Stress hormones may be released, which in turn may negatively affect fetal growth and development and neonatal behavior (Abrams et al 1995, Lundy et al 1998). Stress hormones during pregnancy may negatively impact on birthweight and may lead to preterm labor (Field el al 2004). Deep muscle relaxation has been shown to reduce stress in pregnant adolescents (de Anda et al 1990). Although massage therapy has not been studied as a treatment for the symptoms associated with pregnancy, massage during labor has been shown to decrease labor pain (Field et al 1997). Massage therapy has also been shown to decrease cortisol and chronic lower back pain and to improve sleep patterns (Field et al 1992, Hernandez-Reif et al 1998). In the present study, massage therapy was expected to have a positive impact by decreasing stress hormones and leg and back pain (Field et al 1999).

Method

Participants

Twenty-six pregnant women were recruited during their second trimester and randomly assigned to a massage therapy or progressive muscle relaxation group. The two groups did not differ on demographic variables.

Massage therapy

Starting in their second trimester, participants in the massage group received 10–20-minute massages over 5 weeks (i.e. two massages per week for 5 weeks). The massages were conducted by trained massage therapists. Each session began with the mother in a side-lying position, with pillows positioned behind the back and between the legs for support. The massage was administered in the following sequence for 10 minutes:

1. Head and neck: massaging the scalp, making small circles from the forehead, along the hairline and down to the temple, and kneading the neck from the base up (see Fig. 2.1).
2. Back: using the heel of the hands, moving along the spine; using the palms, moving hands with rocking movements from the top of the shoulder blade to the backbone; pressing fingertips, along both sides of the spine from the neck to the backbone and then stroking upward from the hip to the neck; stroking the shoulder muscles (trapezius); inching up the back, using fingertips placed on sides of the spine, starting from the hipbone to the neck and then reversing direction downward using fingertips in a raking fashion; massaging the lower back from the backbone across the waistline using the heel of the palm to make large circles; long gliding strokes from the hip up and over the shoulder.
3. Arms: making long sweeping strokes from the elbow up and over the shoulder; kneading the muscles from above the elbow to the shoulder;

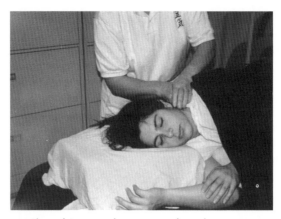

Figure 2.1   Massage therapist massaging a woman's neck.

stroking from the wrist to the elbow; kneading the muscles between the wrist and the elbow.
4. Hands: massaging the hand using thumbs to make small circles to the palm; on the back of the hand, rubbing between the spaces to the bones; sliding down each finger.
5. Legs: long sweeping strokes from the knee to the thigh, up and over the hip; kneading the muscles between the knee and the thigh; long sweeping strokes up and down the calf; kneading of the calf muscle.
6. Feet: massaging the soles from the toes to the heel with fingers and thumbs and moving back towards the toes; sliding down each toe and rotating the toe three times; stroking top of foot towards the leg. The routine was repeated with the mother lying on her other side supported by pillows.

Relaxation therapy

A relaxation group was used for comparison. This group controlled for potential placebo effects or potential improvement related to the increased attention given to the massage group. The relaxation group was given instructions on how to conduct progressive muscle relaxation sessions while lying quietly on the massage table. A session lasted 20 minutes and consisted of tensing and relaxing large muscle groups, starting with the feet and progressing to the calves, thighs, hands, arms, back and face. The participants were asked to conduct these sessions at home twice a week for 5 weeks.

Pre-/post-treatment assessments to measure immediate effects

These assessments were made before and after the sessions on the first and last days of the 5-week study.

State Anxiety Inventory (STAI) (Spielberger et al 1970) This was administered to determine anxiety status. The STAI is comprised of 20 items and assesses how the subject feels at that moment in terms of severity, from 0 = 'not at all' to 4 = 'very much so'. Typical items include 'I feel nervous' and 'I feel calm'. The STAI scores range from 20 to 80 and increase in response to stress and decrease under relaxing conditions.

Profile of Mood States Depression Scale (POMS–D) (McNair et al 1971) The POMS consists of 15 adjectives rating depressed mood 'right now' on a five-point scale ranging from 0 = 'not at all' to 4 = 'extremely', using words such as 'blue' and 'sad'. The scale ranges from 0 to 60.

VITAS (Vitas Healthcare Corporation, FL, USA) Participants completed pre- and post-session pain scales, with reference to leg and back pain, on the first and last day of the study. Pain perception was rated on a visual analog scale (VAS) ranging from 0 = 'no pain' to 10 = 'worst possible pain', and anchored with five faces. The faces, located at two-point intervals, ranged from very happy (0), happy (2), contented (4), somewhat distressed (6), distressed (8), to very distressed (10).

First-/last-day session assessments to measure longer-term effects

On the first and last days of the 5-week study, the following assessments were administered.

Sleep Scale (JA Verran & S Snyder-Halperin, unpublished work, 1986) Questions on this 15-item scale are rated on a visual analog anchored at one end with effective sleep responses (e.g. 'Did not awaken', 'Had no trouble sleeping') and at the opposite end with ineffective responses (e.g. 'Was awake 10 hours', 'Had a lot of trouble falling asleep'). Participants place a mark across the answer line at the point that best reflects their last night's sleep. Higher scores suggest more effective sleep on the effectiveness scale.

Urine samples Urine samples were collected on the first and last days of the study and assayed for cortisol, catecholamines (norepinephrine, epinephrine, dopamine) and serotonin (as 5-HIAA). Based on previous literature, decreased cortisol and catecholamines were expected for the massage group by the end of the 5-week study (Field 1996, Ironson et al 1996).

Obstetric Complications (OCS) and Postnatal Factor (PNF) Scales (Littman & Parmelee 1978) Following delivery, obstetric complications and perinatal factors were quantified using the OCS and PNF scales. The OCS is a 41-item scale that assesses optimality of the prenatal period (e.g. maternal age, medical problems during pregnancy, length of time since last pregnancy), obstetrics (e.g. delivery type, drugs given to mother during labor and delivery, fetal heart rate during labor), and the neonatal period (e.g. placenta previa, onset of stable respiration, Apgar scores). A higher score is optimal and indicates fewer complications. The PNF is a 10-item scale that assesses complications in newborns (e.g. respiratory distress, temperature disturbance, feeding within 48 hours). A higher score is optimal. The OCS and PNF were completed after delivery from information collected from the medical records.

Results

Immediate effects (pre-/post-treatment measures)

Data analyses revealed that self-reported anxiety decreased after the first session for the massage therapy and relaxation groups and after the last session for the massage therapy group (see Table 2.1, Fig. 2.2A). Only the massage therapy group improved in mood from pre- to post-session on the first and last days of the study (Fig. 2.2B). Back pain decreased for the massage therapy group immediately following the first and last sessions and less leg pain occurred for both groups from pre- to post-session on both days (Fig. 2.3).

Longer-term effects (first/last day measures)

Data analyses revealed that less disrupted sleep occurred by the last day of the study for the massage therapy group (change in score from 49 to 38 vs an unchanging score of 50). A significant decrease was noted in norepinephrine levels and an increase in dopamine levels in the massage therapy group across the course of the study (see Table 2.2). The massage therapy group had fewer obstetric complications and their newborns had fewer postnatal complications. Women in the massage therapy group had fewer premature births, and their infants required less ventilatory assistance.

Table 2.1   Means for the massage therapy and relaxation groups for short-term measures (pre-/post-session)

	Massage		Relaxation	
	First day pre-/post-	Last day pre-/post-	First day pre-/post-	Last day pre-/post-
Short-term measures				
STAI (anxiety)	36/23.0	33.9/28.0	38.8/22.8[a]	32.8/30.0
POMS (mood)	1.9/0.6[a]	2.7/0.9[a]	1.8/1.3	2.8/3.0
VITAS				
Back pain	4.6/2.2[a]	3.8/2.1[a]	3.4/3.3	3.2/3.5
Leg pain	2.0/1.2[a]	1.5/0.9[a]	2.3/1.4[a]	3.8/2.6[a]

[a]Significant difference between adjacent numbers: lower scores are optimal.

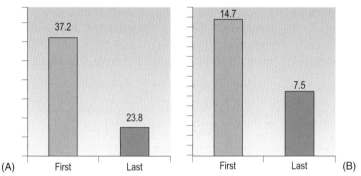

Figure 2.2 Outcomes after massage therapy in (A) pregnancy anxiety, (B) pregnancy depression.

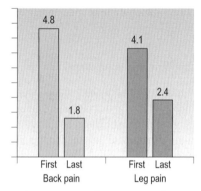

Figure 2.3 Back and leg pain—outcome after massage therapy.

Table 2.2 Means for massage therapy and relaxation group for biochemical measures (first/last day), obstetric and postnatal complications

Variables	Massage First/last day	Relaxation First/last day
Biochemical measures (ng/ml)		
Cortisol	91/185	199/204
Norepinephrine	42/28[a]	35/43
Epinephrine	8/6	3/4
Dopamine[a]	300/399[a]	370/444[a]
Serotonin[a]	4448/4651	3697/3995
Obstetric complications[a]	115.4	95.8[a]
Pre-eclampsia	11%	22%
Prematurity	0%	33%
Postnatal complications[a]	136.2	115.3[a]
Ventilatory	0%	33%[a]

[a]Higher scores/levels are optimal and [a]significant difference between adjacent numbers.

Discussion

The decrease in norepinephrine levels would be expected to positively affect pregnancy outcomes and may have contributed to the lower obstetric (e.g. less prematurity) and postnatal complication scores (e.g. less ventilatory assistance provided to infants) for the massage therapy group. Massage may reduce prematurity via reduced stress hormones (Paarlberg et al 1995). Back and leg pain relief from massage therapy may have also contributed to the massaged women's report of less sleep disturbance, or less sleep disturbance may have contributed to less pain, as was suggested by Sunshine et al (1996) in a massage therapy study on fibromyalgia. Increased dopamine may have some clinical significance for specific pregnancy problems, such as pre-eclampsia. The findings suggest that massage therapy is effective for reducing pregnant women's anxiety levels, stress hormones, sleep disturbance and back pain and for lessening obstetric and postnatal complications.

STUDY 2: EFFECTS OF MASSAGE THERAPY ON DEPRESSED PREGNANT WOMEN

Depressed pregnant women have been noted in recent studies to have elevated cortisol and norepinephrine levels and low levels of dopamine and serotonin (Field 1998, Field et al 2004). They subsequently gave birth to newborns with depression-like symptoms and with elevated cortisol and norepinephrine levels and lower dopamine and serotonin levels like their mothers (Field et al 2004, Lundy et al 1999). Elevated stress hormones during pregnancy may lead to preterm labor and low birthweight (Field et al 2004, Glover et al 1999, Kurki et al 2000, Paarlberg et al 1995, Wadhwa et al 1998).

Massage therapy may serve as an effective intervention for prenatally depressed women inasmuch as it has been noted to help related conditions. For example, massage therapy has decreased postpartum depression (Field et al 1996) as well as depression-related hormones including cortisol and norepinephrine (Field et al 1996).

The pregnancy massage study on non-depressed women described above (Study 1; Field et al 1999) served as a model for the current study. The present study assessed the effects of massage therapy on depressed pregnant women and assessed a more cost-effective form of massage therapy, having the 'significant other' provide the massages instead of massage therapists. In addition, massage therapy effects on fetal activity, which has been notably elevated in fetuses of depressed mothers (Field et al 2004), was assessed. Massage therapy was expected to have positive effects on the prenatally depressed women by decreasing their stress hormones. After massage therapy the women were also expected to have lower anxiety, less leg and back pain and fewer obstetric complications, and their newborns were expected to perform better on the Brazelton Neonatal Behavior Assessment Scale (see Chapter 1 Appendix 1; Brazelton 1984).

In addition, we assessed a theoretical model derived from data suggesting relationships between prenatal maternal mood states and biochemistry, fetal activity and neonatal outcomes (Field et al 2004, Glover et al 1999, Lundy et al 1999, Wadhwa et al 1998) and the effects of massage therapy on these factors (Field et al 1999). In this model massage therapy increases serotonin and in turn decreases cortisol and depression. In addition, serotonin is noted to reduce leg and back pain. The massage therapy is also expected to increase dopamine and, in turn, decrease norepinephrine and anxiety. Ultimately, these two pathways may lead to reduced fetal activity and better neonatal outcome (gestational age, birthweight, performance on the Brazelton Scale) (see Fig. 2.4 for a proposed model).

Method

Participants

Eighty-four depressed pregnant women were recruited from obstetric and gynecology clinics during their second trimester, and randomly assigned to a massage therapy group, a progressive muscle relaxation comparison group or a standard prenatal care only group. A group of 28 non-depressed women were also recruited as a comparison group. The groups did not differ on demographic variables.

Treatments

Massage therapy   Starting in the second trimester, the massage group received two 20-minute massages per week over 16 weeks. Trained massage therapists taught the massage to the 'significant others' of the women, who

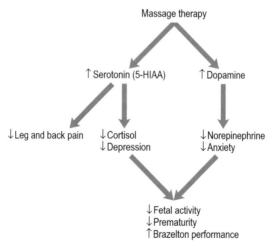

Figure 2.4   Proposed model of effects of pregnancy massage therapy on antenatal and neonatal outcomes.

then conducted the twice-weekly massages for the 16-week period. Each session began with the mother in a side-lying position, with pillows positioned behind her back and between her legs for support. The massage was administered in the following sequence for 10 minutes (Field et al 1999), in the same manner as the previous study, including (1) head and neck, (2) back, (3) arms, (4) hands, (5) legs, and (6) feet. The same routine was repeated once (for a total of 20 minutes) with the mother lying on her other side supported by pillows.

Muscle relaxation   The muscle relaxation group was given instructions on how to conduct progressive muscle relaxation sessions while lying quietly on the massage table. A session lasted 20 minutes and consisted of tensing and relaxing large muscle groups, starting with the feet and progressing to the calves, thighs, hands, arms, back and face. The participants were asked to conduct these sessions at home twice a week for 16 weeks.

Measures

Pre-/post-treatment measures (immediate effects)   These assessments were made before and after the sessions on the first and last days of the 16-week study to document the immediate effects of the therapy, and included the same measures used in the previous study as follows:

- State Anxiety Inventory (STAI) (Spielberger et al 1970)
- Profile of Mood States Scale (POMS) (McNair et al 1971)
- VITAS Pain Scale (VITAS Healthcare Corporation, FL, USA)
- First day/last day session measures (longer-term effects).

On the first and last days of the 16-week study, the following assessments were administered to document longer-term effects of massage therapy. These included the same assessment of urine as made in the previous study as follows: cortisol, norepinephrine, epinephrine, dopamine, and serotonin (as 5-HIAA). In addition, the mothers were given the Center for Epidemiological Studies—Depression (CESD; Radloff 1977) scale, which is a 20-item scale rating depressive symptoms (e.g. 'I feel lonely') over the past week on a four-point scale: 0 = 'rarely', 1 = 'some of the time', 2 = 'occasionally' and 3 = 'most of the time'. Scores range from 0 to 60, with a score >16 being the cutoff point for depression.

Finally, fetal activity was assessed. This assessment was based on the procedure used in an earlier study on maternal depression and fetal activity (Dieter et al 2001) and was made at 18–24 weeks' gestation and again at 36 weeks. Fetal activity was assessed using interval recording on a real-time ultrasound scanner with a single Doppler transducer applied to the mother's abdomen. Every effort was made by the ultrasound technician to visualize the entire fetus. If the fetus could not be fully visualized, the ultrasound technician focused on the head, torso, arms, and upper leg regions, so as to permit the assessment of leg movement. Every 3 seconds, a tape-recorded cue (heard through an earphone) prompted the researcher to record the type of fetal activity occurring when the tone went off. All behavior occurring in-between tones was ignored. The 3-second interval was arbitrarily chosen for its ability to generate an easy total ($60/3 \times 3 = 60$ observations during the 3-minute interval). The researcher recorded: (1) single limb movements, (2) multiple limb movements, (3) gross body movements, (4) no movement. The percentage of the total time that the fetus engaged in each movement category was calculated by taking the total number of movements divided by the total number of observations.

Postnatal variables These included the Obstetric Complications (OCS) and Postnatal Factor (PNF) Scales (Littman & Parmelee 1978) as in the previous study, and the Brazelton Neonatal Behavior Assessment Scale (see Chapter 1/ Appendix; Brazelton 1984). This scale was assessed within a few days after birth. The Brazelton assessments were performed by researchers who were trained to 0.90 reliability and were blind to the group classification of the mothers and infants. This neurobehavioral examination consists of 28 behavior items including responses to a face, voice, and rattle, and self-regulation behaviors, each scored on a nine-point scale, and 20 elicited reflexes, each scored on a three-point scale. The newborn's performance was summarized according to the traditional clusters (Lester et al 1982), and B Lester & E Tronick's (unpublished work, 1992) depression, excitability and withdrawal factors.

Results

Prenatal measures (see Table 2.3)

The data analyses revealed the following:

Table 2.3 Means for maternal prenatal biochemistry on first and last days of the study

Variables	Massage		Relaxation		Depressed control		Non-depressed control	
	First	Last	First	Last	First	Last	First	Last
Cortisol (ng/ml)	328.5[a]	252.2	310.2	294.5	326.0	332.9	271.2	277.0
Norepinephrine (ng/ml)	58.3[a]	46.1	55.4	46.5	52.9	58.7	41.5	47.5
Dopamine (ng/ml)	242.1[a]	274.7	252.9	244.3	289.6	267.8	243.9	260.3
Serotonin (ng/ml)	4247.2[a]	4997.9	3908.6	4284.6	4071.9	4171.9	4822.3	5481.7

[a]Statistically significant difference between first and last day at $p < 0.05$.

- increased serotonin levels
- decreased cortisol levels
- increased dopamine levels
- decreased norepinephrine levels

for the massage therapy group. Because of the increase in serotonin it is not surprising that the massage group experienced a greater decrease in depression on the CES-D and on the Profile of Mood States. A greater improvement in mood and a greater decrease in anxiety were also noted from pre- to post-session for the massage therapy group on the first and last days of the study. Data analyses also showed a greater decrease in fetal activity for the massage group. The massage group had better obstetric complications scale scores than the muscle relaxation group. The factors contributing to the better obstetric complication scores were a lesser incidence of prematurity and low birthweight in the babies of the massaged group. Data analyses revealed decreased back pain for the massage therapy group immediately following the first and last sessions, and lessened leg pain for the massage and relaxation groups from pre-to-post session on the first day and only for the massage therapy group on the last day (see Table 2.4). The increase in serotonin levels may have contributed to decreased leg and back pain.

Postnatal measures

The lesser incidence of prematurity and low birthweight in the massage group may have contributed to massaged neonates' more optimal performance on the Brazelton Scale, including:

- better scores than the control group on the habituation, range of state, autonomic stability, and withdrawal scores
- better scores than both the muscle relaxation and control groups on the depressed scale
- better scores than the control group on the motor maturity scale (see Table 2.5).

Discussion

In the proposed model, massage therapy was expected to lead to increased serotonin (as 5-HIAA) and dopamine. This hypothesis was derived from massage therapy effects data from other studies (see Field 1998 for a review). Serotonin was expected to decrease depression and cortisol, which in turn would be expected to decrease the incidence of premature delivery (Field et al 1999). The increased serotonin and decreased cortisol may have contributed to the better neonatal outcome in this study, providing support for the left pathway of the proposed model (see Fig. 2.1). Elevated serotonin (as 5-HIAA) may have also contributed to the reduced leg and back pain, as serotonin is noted to decrease substance P and other pain-causing chemicals (Moldofsky 1982).

Table 2.4   Means for neonatal variables on first and last days of study

Variables Immediate effects	Massage		Relaxation		Depressed control		Non-depressed control	
	Pre-	Post-	Pre-	Post-	Pre-	Post-	Pre-	Post-
Anxiety (STAI)								
First day	37.4[a]	26.8	45.5	37.5	36.4	34.7	30.3	29.6
Last day	42.0[a]	29.5	44.6	35.4	39.4	36.3	31.4	30.2
Mood (POMS)								
First day	8.4[a]	2.2	9.2	7.4	8.5	7.9	3.1	2.4
Last day	8.2[a]	2.5	9.6	7.3	8.7	9.7	1.5	0.9
Leg pain								
First day	3.1[a]	0.9	2.6	1.7	2.9	2.8	1.4	1.5
Last day	3.6[a]	2.0	3.6	2.6	2.3	2.2	2.3	2.3
Back pain								
First day	3.5[a]	0.8	3.9	3.5	2.3	2.2	1.7	1.7
Last day	2.9[a]	2.0	4.0	3.5	2.6	2.4	1.7	1.8
Longer-term effects	First	Last	First	Last	First	Last	First	Last
CES-D	24.9[a]	19.9	26.2	24.8	28.3	27.8	6.5	8.1
Fetal movement (%)	10.2[a]	1.9	7.9	2.7	7.8	3.5	9.8	3.4
Obstetric complications[a]	102.1		91.2		78.0		105.3	
Postnatal complications[a]	134.9		134.7		113.8		149.4	

[a]Statistical difference between columns at least at $p<0.05$.
[a]Higher scores are optimal.

Massage therapy also contributed to increased dopamine, which has been noted to dampen norepinephrine levels. Norepinephrine and its associated anxiety state (Glover et al 1999) decreased. These, in turn, may have also decreased obstetric complications (prematurity and low birthweight). Dopamine may have reduced other related obstetric complications, as it has been shown to improve renal function (Nasu et al 1996) and urine output in postpartum women with high blood pressure (Mantel & Makin 1997), suggesting that increased dopamine may have some clinical significance for specific pregnancy problems, such as pre-eclampsia. Reduced fetal activity may have also resulted from reduced anxiety and stress hormones (Nasu et al 1996).

Unfortunately, although these data provide empirical evidence for the effects noted in the proposed model, the sample was too small to conduct path analysis to test the relative significance of the pathways. Other limita-

Table 2.5   Means for postnatal variables

	Massage	Relaxation	Depressed control	Non-depressed control
Brazelton				
Habituation	6.4	5.3	4.4	5.7
Orientation	4.1	4.5	3.5	4.9
Motor maturity	4.3	4.4	3.2	5.1
Range of state	3.7	3.4	3.0	3.9
State regulation	4.5	4.7	4.2	4.8
Autonomic stability	6.2	5.9	5.1	6.7
Abnormal reflexes[a]	2.7	4.0	2.5	3.2
Withdrawal[a]	2.7	3.0	4.1	2.2
Excitability[a]	2.3	2.1	2.1	2.7
Depressed[a]	3.6	4.4	5.8	2.6

[a]Lower scores are optimal. See text for statistically significant differences.

tions of the study include the reliance on subjective self-reports and deriving obstetric and postnatal complications data from medical records, which are often inaccurate. Further, a better design would have been a comparison of different forms or intensities of massage. However, it was found that it was too difficult to control or monitor different types or different pressure massages when they were conducted by significant others. Also, although the relaxation group may have been less compliant, the group differences favoring the massage group suggest that at least the significant others were compliant in providing massages. Nonetheless, these data confirm and extend our previous study results (Field et al 1999). Overall, the findings suggest that massage therapy is effective for reducing pregnant women's stress hormones, stressful mood states, leg and back pain, and for lessening obstetric and postnatal complications, hence improving neonatal outcomes. They also suggest the efficacy of using significant others as massage therapists. Further research is needed to explore the underlying mechanisms for these changes.

STUDY 3: FETAL ACTIVITY FOLLOWING STIMULATION OF THE MOTHER'S ABDOMEN, FEET AND HANDS

Vibratory stimulation has been shown to affect fetal activity, although fetal responses to vibratory stimulation are not apparent until about 26 weeks' gestation (Hepper & Shahidullah 1994). At this stage, movement in response to stimulation only occurs at a rate of 60%, increasing to a rate of 80% by 32 weeks' gestation. Despite the wealth of research on vibratory stimulation applied to the mother's abdomen, only a few studies have assessed fetal responses to other external forms of stimulation. Massaging highly innervated areas such as the feet and hands may also stimulate fetal activity. Massaging these areas may evoke neurochemical changes, affect blood flow to the fetus via changes in uterine artery resistance, or both. Massage therapy has been shown, for example, to affect maternal cortisol and catecholamine levels (Field 1998) which may, in turn, affect fetal activity.

We measured the effects of foot massage and hand massage on fetal activity. Foot and hand massage, as opposed to massage on any other body parts, were used because the feet and hands are highly innervated, and fetal responses to maternal foot acupuncture have been noted at late- but not mid-gestation (Cardini & Weixin 1998). We also assessed the fetal response to vibratory stimulation to determine if fetal responses to direct stimulation vs indirect simulation (of the mother's feet and hands) were different. Because the typically applied vibratory stimulus has a duration of only 3 seconds and massages are usually longer in duration, the data were compared to their own controls.

In this study the fetal response to foot massage was assessed. Of concern here was whether fetuses might respond to massage in this highly innervated area (the feet), as the 33-week-old fetuses had responded to acupuncture of the feet in the study by Cardini & Weixin (1998), but at the earlier age of 20 weeks' gestation.

Method

Participants

Forty mothers were recruited during their second trimester (M = 20 weeks' gestation) to receive foot massage.

Procedure

Immediately prior to a standard clinical ultrasound examination, the women were asked to complete an informed consent and a demographic questionnaire. The State Anxiety Inventory (STAI; Spielberger et al 1970) was completed immediately before and after the ultrasound procedure as a measure of relaxation. The mothers were then monitored by ultrasound for fetal activity while lying on an ultrasound examination table in a left recumbent position. All participants were assessed between 10.00am and 2.00pm in the same ultrasound examination office. No significant differences were noted in the assessment times or the days the women were assessed.

The procedures consisted of the observation of fetal activity for a total of 9 minutes while the mothers rested quietly during a 3-minute baseline period, followed by a 3-minute foot massage or control period followed by a 3-minute post-stimulation observation period.

Results and discussion

Fetal movement was greater following the foot massage than following the control condition (see Fig. 2.5). In another comparison, the hands—another

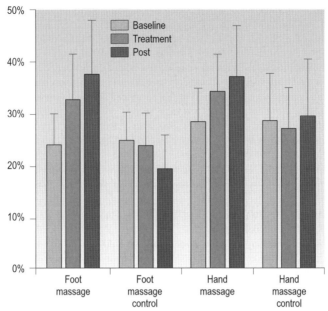

Figure 2.5 Percent time total fetal movement occurred in response to foot and hand massage.

highly innervated area of the body—were stimulated to determine if these findings were specific to the feet, as in this study and in the acupuncture study showing increased fetal activity following stimulation of the feet (Cardini & Weixin 1998). The hands, like the feet, are among the most highly innervated areas of the human body, with numerous connections to the central nervous system and numerous reflex arches (Kandel et al 2000, Nolte 1999). Thus, we expected to find a similar fetal response after stimulation of the mother's hands.

While the hand massage procedure elicited a 10% increase in fetal movement, compared to a 16% increase for the foot massage procedure, this change in fetal activity was not significantly different from that shown by a control group. We expected that fetuses of mothers receiving the hand massage procedure would show a similar response to that of fetuses of mothers receiving a foot massage. Perhaps massaging the hands elicits a less intense physiological response than massaging the feet. Research on the effect of maternal exercise on fetal activity indicates that moderate and strenuous exercise affect the fetus differentially (Manders et al 1997, Marsal et al 1979). While light exercise produces slight or no changes, moderate exercise produces the opposite effect. A future study might compare the effects of foot and hand massage on maternal biochemistry variables. This would help to clarify whether the effect of foot massage on fetal movement could be attributed to change in maternal biochemistry and physiology (i.e. maternal respiration, blood pressure, uterine contraction, etc).

References

Abrams SM, Field T, Scafidi F, et al 1995 Maternal depression effects on infants' Brazelton Scale performance. Infant Mental Health Journal 16:231–237.

Brazelton TB 1984 Neonatal Behavior Assessment Scale. Lippincott, Philadelphia.

Cardini F, Weixin H 1998 Moxibustion for correction of breech presentation: a randomized controlled trial. Journal of the American Medical Association 280:1580–1584.

de Anda D, Darroch P, Davidson M et al 1990 Stress management for pregnant adolescents and adolescent mothers: a pilot study. Child and Adolescent Social Work Journal 7:53–67.

Diego M, Dieter J, Field T, et al 2002 Fetal activity following vibratory stimulation of the mother's abdomen and foot and hand massage. Developmental Psychobiology 41:396–406.

Dieter JNI, Field T, Hernandez-Reif M, et al 2001 Maternal depression and increased fetal activity. Obstetrics 21(5):468–473.

Field T 1998 Massage therapy effects. American Psychologist 53:1270–1281.

Field T, Morrow C, Valdeon C, et al 1992 Massage therapy reduces anxiety in child and adolescent psychiatric patients. Journal of the American Academy of Child and Adolescent Psychiatry 31:125–131.

Field T, Grizzle N, Scafidi F, et al 1996 Massage and relaxation therapies' effects on depressed adolescent mothers. Adolescence 31:903–911.

Field T, Hernandez-Reif M, Taylor S, et al 1997 Labor pain is reduced by massage therapy. Journal of Psychosomatic Obstetrics and Gynecology 18:286–291.

Field T, Hernandez-Reif M, Hart S, et al 1999 Pregnant women benefit from massage therapy. Journal of Psychosomatic Obstetrics and Gynecology 20:31–38.

Field T, Diego M, Dieter J, et al 2004 Prenatal depression effects on the fetus and neonate. Infant Behavior & Development 27:216–229.

Glover V, Teixeira J, Gitau R et al 1999 Mechanisms by which maternal mood in pregnancy may affect the fetus. Contemporary Reviews in Obstetrics and Gynecology 24:1–6.

Heliovaara M 1989 Risk factors for low back pain and sciatica. Annals of Medicine 21:257–264.

Hepper PG, Shahidullah BS 1994 Development of fetal hearing. Archives of Disease in Childhood 71:F81–F87.

Hernandez-Reif M, Dieter J, Field T, et al 1998 Migraine headaches are reduced by massage therapy. The International Journal of Neuroscience 96:1–11.

Ironson G, Field T, Scafidi F, et al 1996 Massage therapy is associated with enhancement of the immune system's cytotoxic capacity. The International Journal of Neuroscience 84:205–217.

Kandel ER, Schwartz JH, Jessel TM 2000 Principles of neural science, 4th edn. McGraw-Hill, Columbus, OH.

Kurki T, Hiilesmaa V, Raitasalo R, et al 2000 Depression and anxiety in early pregnancy and risk for preeclampsia. Obstetrics and Gynecology 95:487–490.

Lester B, Als H, Brazelton TB 1982 Regional obstetric anesthesia in newborn behavior: a reanalysis toward synergistic effects. Child Development 53:687–692.

Littman D, Parmelee A 1978 Medical correlates of infant development. Pediatrics 61:470–482.

Lundy B, Jones N, Field T, et al 1998 Prenatal depression effects on neonates. Infant Behavior & Development 22(1):119–129.

Lundy BL, Jones NA, Field T, et al 1999 Prenatal depression effects on neonates. Infant Behavior and Development 22:121–137.

McNair DM, Lorr M, Droppleman LF 1971 POMS—Profile of Mood States. Educational and Industrial Testing Service, San Diego, CA.

Manders MAM, Sonder GJB, Mulder EJH, et al 1997 The effects of maternal exercise on fetal heart rate and movement patterns. Early Human Development 48:237–247.

Mantel GD, Makin JD 1997 Low dose dopamine in postpartum pre-eclamptic women with oliguria: a double-blind, placebo controlled, randomised trial. British Journal of Obstetrics and Gynaecology 104:1180–1183.

Marsal K, Lofgran O, Genser G 1979 Fetal breathing movements and maternal exercise. Acta Obstetrica Gynecologia Scandinavica 58:197–201.

Moldofsky H 1982 Rheumatic pain modulation syndrome: the interrelationships between sleep, central nervous system, serotonin, and pain. Advances in Neurology 33:51–57.

Nasu K, Yoshimatsu J, Anai T, et al 1996 Low-dose dopamine in treating acute renal failure caused by preeclampsia. Gynecologic and Obstetric Investigation 42:140–141.

Nolte J 1999 The human brain, 4th edn. Mosby, St Louis, MO.

Paarlberg K, Vingerhoets A, Passchier J, et al 1995 Psychosocial factors and pregnancy outcome: a review with emphasis on methodological issues. Journal of Psychosomatic Research 39:563–595.

Radloff L 1977 The CES-D scale: a self-report depression scale for research in the general population. Applied Psychological Measurement 1:385–401.

Spielberger CD, Gorsuch RC, Lushene RE 1970 The State Trait Anxiety Inventory. Consulting Psychologists Press, Palo Alto, CA.

Sunshine W, Field T, Quintino O, et al 1996 Fibromyalgia benefits from massage therapy and transcutaneous electrical stimulation. Journal of Clinical Rheumatology 2:18–22.

Wadhwa PD, Porto M, Garite TJ, et al 1998 Maternal corticotropin-releasing hormone levels in the early third trimester predict length of gestation in human pregnancy. American Journal of Obstetrics and Gynecology 179:1079–1085.

Chapter 3

Enhancing growth and development

At least a dozen studies from around the world have now established that preterm infants gain more weight after being given a period of massage therapy during their hospital stay (Field et al 2004). Others have also documented an increase in bone mineralization, bone density, bone length and increased head circumference (Moyer-Mileur et al 1995). Other studies have documented the positive effects of massage therapy on full-term infants, including less irritability and less sleep disturbance (Field et al 1996). The challenge for this field of research is to find potential underlying mechanisms that may be contributing to these growth effects and changes in behavior so that massage therapy might be adopted into hospital practice for preterm and full-term infants. In addition, finding cost-effective ways to deliver the massage, for example teaching the parents infant massage, may enhance the possibility of massage therapy being adopted into practice.

In this chapter, studies on underlying mechanisms and parent delivery of massage are reviewed. In the first study we were able to demonstrate a more cost-effective massage therapy, that is that massage therapy had positive effects on weight gain in preterm infants after only 5 days of therapy as opposed to the 10-day therapy period that had been used by researchers previously (Dieter et al 2003). In the second study we report enhanced vagal activity and gastric motility in preterm infants receiving massage therapy (Diego et al 2003). The vagus (one of the 12 cranial nerves) is noted to have extensive branches to various organs in the body, including the gastrointestinal tract. It is thought that the gastrointestinal system is affected by the vagus in two ways. The vagus is thought to help release food absorption hormones such as glucose and insulin and to stimulate gastric motility or movement of the gut wall to facilitate food absorption. In this study we reported that vagal activity and gastric motility were both enhanced by massage therapy, which, in turn, would be expected to contribute to the weight gain in preterm infants. In Study 3, we report the results of research in which parents delivered the massage to their full-term newborns from day 1 to the end of the first month (Field et al 2004). Here we found that those infants gained more weight and gained more length as well as performing better on the Brazelton Neonatal Behavior Assessment Scale by the end of the month. This study highlighted the potential cost-effectiveness of parents rather than therapists delivering the massage. Parents could be taught by massage therapists in infant massage classes, and then the parents could continue the massages at home. In Study 4, we again taught parents to deliver the massage therapy, but this time with infants and toddlers, in an attempt to reduce sleep disturbances (Field & Hernandez-Reif 2001). Massage therapy was once again shown to be effective in reducing sleep disturbances.

STUDY 1: STABLE PRETERM INFANTS GAIN MORE WEIGHT AND SLEEP LESS AFTER 5 DAYS OF MASSAGE THERAPY

A number of studies have shown that the 10-day massage therapy protocol introduced by Field and colleagues (1986) promotes weight in preterm infants (Ferber et al 2002, Jinon 1996, Kuhn et al 1991, Scafidi et al 1986, 1990, Wheeden et al 1993). The average daily weight gain in these studies was 28–47% greater in the massage groups, despite similar formula and caloric intake.

The 10-day massage therapy protocol also alters the distribution of sleep and awake states. Across studies, the massaged preterm infants spent more time in active alertness and showed better performance on the Brazelton exam at the end of the treatment period (Field et al 1987, Scafidi et al 1986, 1990, Wheeden et al 1993). Furthermore, the massaged preterm infants were discharged between 3 and 6 days sooner than the control infants, accounting for lower hospital costs.

In the first 10-day massage study, Field and colleagues (1996) suggested that the weight gain advantage for the massage group first emerged after 5 days of treatment. The goal of the current study was to examine the effects of 5 days of massage therapy on the weight gain and sleep/awake behavior of preterm infants. Showing that an abbreviated protocol is beneficial warrants the continued use of massage therapy for hospitalized preterm infants who are being discharged earlier from intermediate care nurseries and at lighter weights.

Method

Participants

A random stratification procedure was used to assign infants to either the massage therapy group (n = 16) or the control group (n = 16). All infants were medically stable and were not receiving i.v. fluids, oxygen, phototherapy, antibiotics, or gavage feeds at the start of the study.

Procedure

The massage therapy protocol used by Field et al (1986) was also used for this study. Massage therapy was begun on the day following the study assignment, and it was continued for 5 consecutive days. As in previous studies, the first 15-minute massage occurred approximately 1 hour after the morning feeding, the second about 30 minutes after the midday feeding, and the third approximately 45 minutes after the completion of the second stimulation period.

Each treatment session consisted of 5 minutes of tactile stimulation, followed by 5 minutes of kinesthetic stimulation, and concluded with another 5-minute period of tactile stimulation. The therapists warmed their hands prior to the start of treatment and remained silent during the 15-minute interval.

During tactile stimulation, the infant was placed in a prone position and was given moderate-pressure stroking with the flats of the fingers of both hands. Five 1-minute intervals, consisting of six 10-second periods of stroking, were applied to the following body regions: (1) from the top of the infant's head, down the back of the head to the neck and back to the top of the head; (2) from the back of the neck across the shoulders and back to the neck; (3) from the upper back down to the buttocks and returning to the upper back (contact with the spine was avoided); (4) simultaneously on both legs from the hips to the feet and back to the hips; and (5) both arms simultaneously from the shoulders to the wrists.

For the kinesthetic phase, the infant was placed in a supine position (Fig. 3.1). Each of the five 1-minute segments consisted of six passive flexion/extension movements lasting approximately 10 seconds each. These 'bicycling-like' movements of the limbs occurred in the following sequence: (1) right arm; (2) left arm; (3) right leg; (4) left leg; (5) both legs simultaneously. Nursing notes were examined daily for weight gain.

Sleep/awake behaviors were coded via live observations at the same time on the pre-assignment and last days of the study. That both observations

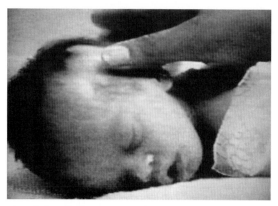

Figure 3.1   Premature infant being massaged.

occurred at the same time controlled the potential effects that circadian rhythm or environmental factors (e.g. reduced lighting at night) have on preterm infant behaviors. Furthermore, day 5 observations occurred approximately 90 minutes after the day's first massage, thus allowing sufficient time for any immediate treatment effects on behavior to subside. A standardized behavior coding system was used that included the following states: (1) non-REM sleep; (2) active sleep without REM; (3) REM sleep; (4) drowsy; (5) quiet alert; (6) active alert; (7) crying (Thoman 1975). The 30-minute observations were recorded on a laptop computer using a program that records the percent time (% time) the infant spent in each behavior state. Observers were trained to 85% interrater-agreement.

Results and discussion

On average the massage therapy group gained 26 g more per day than the control group, suggesting a 53% greater average daily weight gain (see Fig. 3.2). The massage group also spent less time sleeping on the last day than the control group (53% vs 81%), which can be viewed as a positive effect, possibly reflecting acceleration in the developmental course of sleep/wake patterns in preterm infants.

STUDY 2: VAGAL ACTIVITY, GASTRIC MOTILITY AND WEIGHT GAIN IN MASSAGED PRETERM NEONATES

The question of how massage therapy facilitates weight gain in preterm infants remains unanswered. One hypothesis was that massage leads infants to consume more calories. However, preterm infants who received massage did not consume more formula or calories than the control preterm infants (Dieter et al 2003, Ferber et al 2002, Field et al 1986, Jinon 1996, Scafidi et al 1990, Wheeden et al 1993). A second hypothesis was that massaged infants saved more calories by sleeping more. However, the massaged infants were

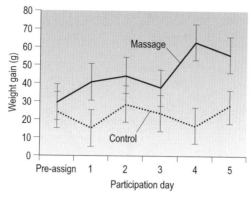

Figure 3.2 Mean weight gain (g) across 5-day massage therapy study for preterm infants.

more alert and spent more time in active awake states than control infants, suggesting that enhanced weight gain was not achieved by saved calories (Scafidi et al 1990).

A third and more favored hypothesis is that moderate-pressure massage stimulates vagal activity, with the vegetative branch of the vagus facilitating the release of food absorption hormones, such as insulin, and increasing gastric motility, leading to more efficient food absorption (Field 1988). This hypothesized mechanism is based on our own work showing increased vagal activity and insulin levels in preterm infants following massage therapy (Field 1988), on the rat data of Saul Schanberg, showing that moderate-pressure stroking is critical for stimulating the release of ornithine decarboxylase (ODC; an index of growth hormone; Pauk et al 1986, Schanberg & Field 1987), and the data of Uvnas-Moberg et al (1987) in both the rat and human models, showing that stimulation of pressure receptors in the intra-oral cavity increases vagal activity and the release of food absorption hormones.

The present study examined this potential mechanism by assessing indices of vagal activity and gastric activity in preterm newborns receiving massage therapy. Based on previous findings we expected that preterm infants receiving massage therapy would show greater weight gain and vagal activity (during the treatment period) than control infants. Furthermore, based on our proposed model (Fig. 3.3) we expected that the moderate-pressure massage therapy would lead to greater vagal activity, gastric activity and weight gain during the massage therapy but not the sham therapy sessions.

Method

Participants

Our sample was comprised of 48 preterm infants recruited from a neonatal intensive care unit. Infants were distributed 44% male, and 46% were African-American, 43% Hispanic and 11% Caucasian. Their mean gestational age was

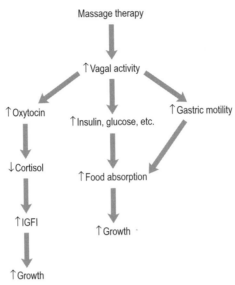

Figure 3.3 Proposed model for weight gain.

29.9 weeks, and they weighed an average 1180 g at birth and 1483 g at study entry. The groups did not differ on these and other background variables.

Procedure

Following informed consent from the parents and attending physician, 54 hospitalized preterm infants were stratified based on birthweight and then randomly assigned to a control (n = 19), massage therapy (n = 18), or sham massage therapy group (n = 17). All participants continued to receive standard nursery care during the course of the study. Data collection was conducted by researchers blind to the group assignment. Electrocardiograms (ECGs) and electrogastrograms (EGGs) were collected on the first day of the study. Physiological data were collected for a total of 45 minutes (15 minutes baseline, 15 minutes treatment and 15 minutes post-treatment).

Treatment Treatment was provided for three 15-minute periods per day for 5 days, approximately 1 hour after feeding, by massage therapists trained on the protocol, who played no other role in the study and who were blind to the hypotheses of the study. The massage therapy consisted of the 15-minute preterm infant massage therapy protocol used by Field et al (1986). The sham massage followed the same protocol. The scheduling and duration of the sham massage sessions were identical to the massage therapy sessions except light-pressure stroking was used during the first and last 5-minute periods of the procedure. The middle 5-minute period of kinesthetic stimulation remained the same.

ECG   A 45-minute ECG recording was collected from each infant on the first and last days of the study to derive measures of heart rate. ECGs were acquired by placing three disposable electrodes on the preterm infants' chest and back.

EGG   A 45-minute EGG recording was collected from each infant on the first and last days of the study to assess gastric activity. EGGs were acquired by placing a ground electrode and two disposable silver chloride electrodes on the preterm infants' abdomen and back.

Results

Preterm infants in the massage therapy (18–35 g/day), but not the control (21–24 g/day) or sham massage groups (25–28 g/day) gained significantly more weight during the treatment period than during the baseline period. A significant trend for only the massage therapy group indicated significantly greater than baseline cardiac vagal tone values during and after the massage therapy sessions (see Figs 3.4 and 3.5). An increase in gastric activity and a decrease in tachygastria occurred for only the massage therapy group. Change in weight gain was significantly related to vagal tone for the moderate-pressure massage therapy group. Change in vagal tone was significantly related to gastric activity during the treatment, suggesting that increased vagal activity led to increased gastric activity. Similarly, the change in gastric activity post-treatment was related to weight gain.

Discussion

Field (2001) proposed a potential mechanism underlying these effects, including that moderate-pressure massage activated the vagus nerve, in turn releas-

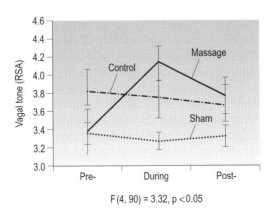

$$F\,(4, 90) = 3.32, p < 0.05$$

Figure 3.4   Cardiac vagal tone 15 minutes before, during and after treatment.

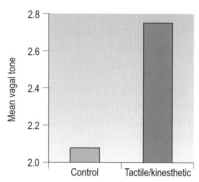

Figure 3.5   Mean vagal tone across massage therapy and control subjects.

ing food absorption hormones and increasing gastric activity, leading to weight gain. In the current sample, vagal activity peaked during the massage therapy period and remained significantly higher than baseline throughout the 15-minute post-stimulation period. Preterm infants receiving massage therapy did not exhibit increased cardiac sympathetic index activity during or after the massage therapy procedure. Thus, massage therapy did not result in autonomic nervous system arousal. As expected, increased gastric activity and decreased tachygastria were observed during the treatment and post-treatment periods.

These moderate- vs light-pressure massage findings suggest the involvement of pressure receptors and/or baroreceptors. Animal studies also indicate that pressure receptor stimulation activates the vagus, in turn, releasing food absorption hormones (Uvnas-Moberg et al 1987) and ODC (Pauk et al 1986, Schanberg & Field 1987). Further, a recent study indicated that compared to light-pressure stimulation, moderate-pressure stimulation reduced heart rate and central nervous system arousal in adults (Diego et al 2003), and an infant massage study indicated more optimal growth and development across the first few months following moderate- vs light-pressure massage (Field et al 2004). Consistent with our model, the change in vagal activity elicited by massage therapy was significantly related to gastric activity. Vagal activation was related to gastric activity, and both vagal tone and gastric activity were, in turn, related to average daily weight gain across the 5-day treatment interval. This suggests that infants who show an increase in vagal activity and gastric activity are more likely to benefit from massage therapy. In fact, the 12 preterm infants who showed an increase rather than a decrease in vagal activity during the massage gained on average over twice as many grams (18 g vs 8 g) during treatment compared to baseline than the four infants who exhibited a decrease in vagal activity.

Taken together, these findings provide strong support for our hypothesized model (Fig. 3.6), indicating that moderate-pressure massage results in increased vagal activity, which, in turn, results in enhanced gastric activity (and potentially the release of food absorption hormones) leading to the

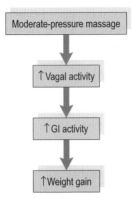

Figure 3.6   Potential model for effect of massage therapy on growth.

greater weight gain that has been consistently observed across preterm infant massage studies.

STUDY 3: MASSAGE THERAPY BY PARENTS IMPROVES EARLY GROWTH AND DEVELOPMENT

Massage therapy facilitates the growth and development of healthy preterm infants (Field et al 1986). A meta-analysis of 19 stimulation studies on preterm infants suggests that 72% of the infants who received massage showed greater weight gain and development relative to control infants who received standard treatment but no additional stimulation (Ottenbacher et al 1987). In a study on full-term infants conducted by Field et al (1996), 40 full-term 1- to 3-month-old infants born to depressed adolescent mothers who were low socioeconomic status (SES) and single parents were given 15 minutes of either massage or rocking for 2 days per week for a 6-week period. The infants who experienced massage therapy spent more time in active alert and active awake states, cried less, and had lower saliva cortisol levels compared to infants in the rocking group, suggesting lower stress. After the sessions, the infants spent less time in an active awake state, suggesting that massage may be more effective than rocking for inducing sleep. Over the 6-week period, the massage therapy infants gained more weight, showed greater improvement on emotionality, sociability, and soothability temperament dimensions and had greater decreases in urine stress hormones. These results were more positive than those of earlier studies, perhaps because of the use of moderate pressure. The earlier studies had used light stroking because of the concern for the delicacy of the infant's skin.

Only a handful of studies have investigated the differential effects of light-pressure versus moderate-pressure massage. Moderate-pressure massage, in contrast to light-pressure stroking, has been shown to have significant psychological and physiological effects. In one study, moderate-pressure stroking increased both range of motion and skin resistance, decreased mean heart rate and electromyography and caused changes in electroneuromyography, whereas no such effects occurred for light-pressure stroking (McKechnie et al 1983). In addition, a study of alpha motor neuron excitability demonstrated that moderate-pressure massage reduced H-reflex excitability, while light-fingertip pressure did not have this effect (Sullivan et al 1991). Light pressure, moreover, has been found to have no effects on limb blood flow as shown by a Doppler ultrasound (Shoemaker et al 1997).

The present study investigated the effects of moderate- and light-pressure massage on the growth and development of infants through the first month of life. Based on previous findings, we expected that infants in the moderate-pressure group would show a greater increase in weight and body length as well as better performance on the Brazelton scale from birth to 1 month of age than infants who received light-pressure massage. Finally, we expected that infants in the moderate-pressure massage group, as opposed to infants in the light-pressure group, would exhibit less agitated behavior during sleep.

Method

Participants

The sample was comprised of 104 full-term newborns (M gestational age = 39 weeks) who were randomly assigned to receive moderate-pressure massage or light-pressure massage. Eight infants did not complete the study (four in each group), yielding a final sample of 96 infants. The infants in both groups were normal birthweight. The groups did not differ on demographic or birth measures.

Procedure

Massage therapy   Soon after the birth of their infants, mothers visited our laboratory where they were taught how to massage their infants and instructed to do so once per day before bedtime. Each massage session consisted of 5 minutes of stroking the infant in a prone position (i.e. six 10-second strokes to the head, shoulders, back, legs, and arms) using either moderate pressure or light pressure, followed by 5 minutes of 10-second extensions and flexions of arms (individually) and legs (individually and together), and concluding with another 5-minute period of stroking as in the first 5-minute stroking segment. To let the mothers know how much pressure to apply, the mothers of dark-skinned infants were shown how the skin was slightly indented by the moderate pressure, and the mothers of light-skinned infants were told about the slight indentation as well as a slight color change accompanying the moderate pressure. To assess compliance, the mothers recorded their massage times on a calendar, and those were periodically checked. However, compliance was easier to assess by simply watching the mothers demonstrate the massage prior to the assessments. Compliance was indicated by the expertise with which they demonstrated the massage for us.

Assessments

Growth measures   Infants' weight was obtained by weighing the mother on an adult weight scale first with and then without her infant, and taking the difference of the mother–infant combined weight and the mother's weight. To record the length, infants were placed with one leg extended on a massage table in a prone position. A mark was drawn on the paper sheet under the infant at both the base of the head and heel, and then the distance between the two marks was measured using a cloth measuring tape. The head circumference was obtained by wrapping the measuring tape around the infant's head at the level of the occipital bone and the center of the forehead.

The Brazelton Neonatal Behavior Assessment Scale (BNBAS) (Brazelton 1973)   This scale was administered at birth and at 1 month of age. The scale is comprised of 20 neurological reflex items and 27 other items summarized according to seven factors: habituation, orientation, motor behavior, range of state, state regulation, autonomic stability and abnormal reflexes (Lester et al 1982). In addition, robustness, excitability and depressive behavior were recorded. The Brazelton examiners were unaware of the infants' group assignments and were trained to a 0.90 reliability criterion prior to the study.

Sleep/wake behavior   To determine the effects of the therapy on sleep/wake behavior, the infants were observed by a researcher during 45-minute sessions on the first and last days of the study period. The observer recorded the infant's predominant state and sleep/wake behaviors using a time-sampling unit methodology with 10-second recording intervals (Guthertz & Field 1989). The total time-sample units were converted to percentage observation time that different states and behaviors occurred for the purposes of data analyses.

Results

The data analyses were conducted on the measures taken on the first and last days of the study, including weight gain, length, head circumference, Brazelton scale performance and sleep/wake measures. The moderate-pressure massage therapy group showed a significantly greater increase than the light-massage therapy group in weight and in length from birth to 1 month of age (see Table 3.1). Significantly improved performance on the Brazelton scale occurred for the moderate-pressure massage therapy group vs the light-pressure massage therapy group as follows: (1) orientation scores increased; (2) excitability scores decreased for the moderate-pressure massage group and increased significantly for the light-pressure massage therapy group; (3) the moderate-pressure massage therapy group received significantly lower scores on the Brazelton depression scale by the end of the first month (see Table 3.2).

Sleep/wake behavior changes favoring the moderate- vs the light-pressure massage therapy group by the end of the study included the following (see Table 3.3): (1) REM sleep decreased more for the moderate- than the light-

Table 3.1   Means for growth measures at birth and 1 month for moderate- and light-pressure massage therapy groups

	Massage group			
	Moderate		Light	
	Birth	1 month	Birth	1 month
Weight (lbs)	7.5	10.0[a]	7.9	9.9
Length (cm)	50.2	53.2[a]	51.6	53.9
Head circumference (cm)	34.9	36.6	34.9	36.0

[a]Significant differences between columns.

Table 3.2   Mean Brazelton scores at birth and 1 month for moderate- and light-pressure massage therapy groups

	Massage group			
	Moderate		Light	
	Birth	1 month	Birth	1 month
Habituation	6.0	5.2	5.9	5.4
Orientation	4.0	5.7[a]	5.2	5.7
Motor	5.3	5.3	5.1	5.2
Range of state	3.6	3.9	3.4	3.4
Regulation of state	4.5	5.6	4.6	5.3
Autonomic response	5.7	5.4	6.3	6.4
Reflexes	2.1	2.7	2.1	2.9
Withdrawn	3.0	2.6	3.0	2.6
Excitability	2.4	2.1[a]	1.7	2.8[a]
Depression	2.8	1.8[a]	2.5	2.5

[a]Significant differences between columns.

Table 3.3   Means for sleep measures for moderate- and light-pressure massage therapy groups at birth and 1 month

	Moderate		Light	
	Birth	1 month	Birth	1 month
Deep sleep	35.2	33.3	41.9	40.8
Light sleep	19.9	21.3	18.5	17.6
REM sleep	14.6	7.9[a]	15.1	11.6
Drowsy	17.8	15.5	6.2	7.6
Alert	4.1	5.0	5.6	5.6
Agitated	5.3	2.9[a]	6.8	9.1
Fussy/crying	3.6	3.0	1.7	5.2[a]
Gross movement	19.6	16.1[a]	14.1	18.4[a]

[a]Significant differences between columns.

pressure massage therapy group; (2) agitated behavior decreased for the moderate-pressure massage therapy group and increased for the light-pressure massage therapy group; (3) fussy/crying behavior increased for the light-pressure massage therapy group, while that behavior did not change for the moderate-pressure massage therapy group; and (4) gross movement during sleep observations decreased for the moderate-pressure massage therapy group, while gross movement increased for the light-pressure massage therapy group.

Discussion

The improved orienting scores of the infants who received moderate- vs light-pressure massage therapy are consistent with our data on adults showing EEG changes that conformed to a pattern of heightened alertness (Field et al 1996). In that same study, improved performance on mathematical tasks (less time required and fewer errors) accompanied the EEG pattern of alertness in the same adults receiving massage. Moderate-pressure massage therapy was also associated with lower depression scores in this study. Light-pressure massage therapy, in contrast, was associated with increased excitability scores on the Brazelton scale and increased agitated and fussy behavior as well as increased gross movement during sleep, suggesting greater arousal. These findings are consistent with those reported by Diego et al (2003) on adults who received light-pressure massage. The light-pressure massage group showed increased arousal as indicated by increased heart rate and changes in EEG including decreased delta and increased beta activity, both indicating greater arousal.

The infants in the moderate-pressure massage therapy group showed greater weight gain, which is consistent with the weight gain of the massaged infants of depressed mothers (Field et al 1996). The infants who received moderate- vs light-pressure massage therapy also showed a significantly greater increase in body length from birth to the end of the study, consistent with data reported by Moyer-Mileur et al (1995). We have speculated that the underlying mechanism for the moderate-pressure massage/weight gain relationship is that pressure receptors are stimulated which leads to increased vagal activity which, in turn, stimulates gastric motility and the release of food-absorption hormones in the gastrointestinal tract, a phenomenon that we have reported in other studies (Field 2001). We have also speculated that there may be some growth hormone secretion effects (which we are currently testing in a study on increased IGF1 resulting from massage therapy) and that the release of food-absorption hormones leads to greater metabolic efficiency (see Fig. 3.5).

STUDY 4: SLEEP PROBLEMS IN INFANTS DECREASE FOLLOWING MASSAGE THERAPY

Sleep problems, including difficulty falling asleep (sleep latency longer than 30 minutes) and nighttime waking (waking parents more than once during the night), are the most common problems of infants and toddlers. 23% of children in a pediatric clinic experienced difficulties falling asleep (Salzarulo & Chevalier 1983). As many as 46% of those who experienced disturbances in the first year had difficulties falling asleep later. Some 21% of those with sleep disturbances later failed one or more years at school.

Massage therapy has been shown to be effective in facilitating sleep in at least two studies, one on infants of depressed mothers (Field et al 1996), and one on children and adolescents with psychiatric problems (Field et al 1992). In the study on infants, the latency to sleep decreased from 21 to 9 minutes following 1 month of twice-weekly massages (Field et al 1996). In the study on children and adolescents, lower anxiety and depression levels, less anxious and fidgeting behaviors, lower activity levels and lower pulse and stress hormone levels (saliva cortisol and norepinepherine) and increased nighttime sleep were noted by the end of the study (Field et al 1992).

The purpose of the current study was to assess the effectiveness of the massage therapy in infants and toddlers who had sleep problems (Field & Hernandez-Reif 2001). Although this is a shift from trying to help children to fall asleep unassisted, the considerable physical contact in massage therapy may explain its facilitation of sleep in previous studies. Massage therapy was taught to the parents who then massaged their child just prior to bedtime. While infant massage therapists have anecdotally noted the positive effects of massage on sleep disturbances in infants and young children (McClure 1989), these effects have not been documented. The massage therapy, however, was expected to reduce sleep-delay behaviors and the latency to sleep as well as increase daytime alertness, activity and positive affect.

Method

Participants

Twenty-three infants/toddlers with sleep onset problems participated in this study. The children were recruited from the enrolment lists of university infant/toddler centers that served 8-month- to 3-year-old children. The inclusion criterion was sleep onset problems recorded for at least two of four nights in a bedtime behavior diary. Sleep onset problems were defined as an average sleep onset latency of over 30 minutes and/or disruptive behavior at bedtime, which had become a regular source of stress for the primary caregiver.

Based on a random stratification procedure to ensure group equivalence on gender, ethnicity and child's age, the children were assigned to the massage therapy group or an attention control reading group. The two groups did not differ on the above variables. The massage therapy group consisted of 12 children (7 girls) who received a 15-minute massage from a parent immediately prior to bedtime for 4 weeks. The control group children (11 children; 6 girls) were read a Dr Seuss story by a parent for 15 minutes prior to bedtime for 4 weeks. Assessments were made on the first and last days of the study.

Procedure

Massage therapy   Massage therapists taught the massage to the parents (Fig. 3.7; Field et al 1986). The massage consisted of carefully-timed stroking movements divided into two standardized phases for a total of 15 minutes (first phase: 8 minutes, second phase: 7 minutes). Parents were given a video-tape and written instructions on the massage to use at home as a reference. The first phase began with the child face-up. After stroking the child's face, oil was applied to the legs, and each leg was massaged using long 'milking' strokes (squeezing and twisting strokes) applied from the hip to the ankle. The thumbs were used to massage the bottom of the foot and to make small circles over the ankle and the top of the foot. The leg was again massaged with long milking strokes and then rolled between the hands from the child's knee to ankle. The stomach was massaged for 1 minute, starting with the sides of the hand moving in a paddlewheel fashion, hand over hand, from the diaphragm to the waist. Then, using a circular motion, the flats of the fingers

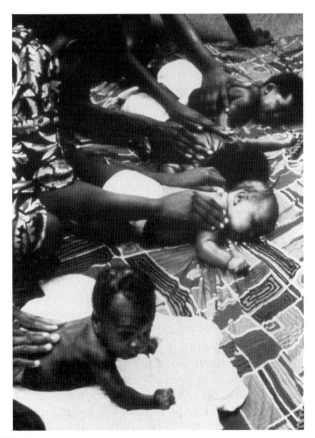

Figure 3.7   Infant massage.

were moved in a clockwise direction and followed with the flats of the hands. The chest was massaged for 1 minute, starting with stroking both sides of the chest, one side at a time, with the flats of the fingers, moving from the middle outward. The flats of the hands were then used with altering cross strokes from the center of the chest and going over the shoulders and then moving both hands simultaneously from the center of the chest to over the shoulders. The arms were massaged, one at a time, each arm for 1 minute following the same procedure as the legs. Finally, the flats of the fingers were used to stroke along the jaw and to massage the nose, cheeks, jaw, chin, and behind the ears. Small firm circles with the flats of the fingers were used to massage the scalp.

Reading group This group was read a Dr Seuss story by a parent for 15 minutes prior to bedtime for 4 weeks. The reading group was included as an attention control group.

Instructions to parents Parents were given written instructions for bedtime rituals (Ferber 1985). They were asked to put the child in bed at a regular time and, as much as possible, not to vary from that time. They were asked to record the usual pre-bed grooming and washing procedures in order to perform this in the same order every night. After placing the child in the child's bed, parents were instructed then either to read a story or to give the child a massage for 15 minutes. Afterwards, parents tucked the child in, said goodnight, turned on a night-light (if used), turned off the lights, and then left the room. Parents were instructed to refrain from entering the child's room for at least 5 minutes if the child cried, and for increasingly longer periods of time, increasing in 5-minute intervals each time. If parents felt compelled to go into the child's room, they were asked to keep both the time in the room and the communication with the child to a minimum. Parents were requested not to lay on the child's bed or to let the child sleep on the parent's bed. Although both groups of parents reported only very occasional incidence of sleeping together, it is possible that this instruction meant that the children, particularly the reading group children, were receiving less physical contact than usual during this study.

Measures

Bedtime behavior diary This diary was developed specifically for this study. For the child's bedtime behavior data, parents (1) circled the behaviors that their children displayed before going to sleep (e.g. asking for a glass of water, crying or calling parents, getting out of bed, standing up in crib, etc.), (2) estimated the length of bedtime preparation, and (3) time until the child fell asleep (in minutes). Then, parents (1) rated how difficult it was to get their child to sleep on a 5-point Likert Scale from 1 = very difficult to 5 = very easy, (2) rated how they felt about the night's bedtime on a 5-point Likert Scale from 1 = very anxiously stressed to 5 = very relaxed, (3) rated the child's bedtime activity level on a 5-point Likert Scale from 1 = very active to 5 = not active at all, (4) compared the night's bedtime behavior to baseline from 1 = very easy to 5 = very difficult, and (5) rated the ease with which the child fell asleep from 1 = very easy to 5 = very difficult. In addition, the parents indicated if the child had had any difficulty falling asleep on any nights during the past week.

Sleep/wake behavior observations   To provide a more objective observation by an observer (a psychology graduate student) who was blind to the children's group assignment, subjects were also observed at their nursery school at 2 pm for a 45-minute period on the first and last afternoons of the intervention period. Thoman's (1975) coding system was used to record sleep/wake states that naturally occurred at the time. Thoman's coding system includes non-REM sleep, active sleep, REM sleep, drowsy, alert inactivity, awake activity and fussing/crying states that are recorded at 10-second intervals. In addition, as a general measure of activity level and affect, the presence of multiple limb movements (more than one limb moving at a time), mouthing and smiling were recorded.

Results

Data analysis revealed that children in the massage therapy group showed fewer bedtime disruptive behaviors and a shorter latency to sleep (see Table 3.4). Parents who massaged their child reported less difficulty getting their child to sleep, less anxiety about putting their child to sleep, improved bedtime behaviors, and greater ease of going to sleep for their child. Data analysis comparing the two groups on their nursery school sleep/wake behaviors on the first and last days of the study (see Table 3.5) suggested that the massage therapy versus the storytelling group spent less time in deep and active sleep during the behavior observations by the end of the study, more time in alert inactive and alert active states, more time showing multiple limb movements, less time mouthing, and more time smiling (see Table 3.5).

Discussion

Organized activities, as in the current study, may reduce the length of bedtime preparation. Both reading stories and massage therapy, according to the parents in this study, reduced the length of bedtime preparation and the children's activity level. Massage therapy may be particularly effective at reducing sleep problems. For example, in a previous study, children who had been hospitalized for psychiatric problems spent more time in nighttime sleep, with fewer night-wakings, following 1 week of daily massages (Field et al 1992). In the current study fewer of the massaged children had problems falling asleep and that group of children had shorter latency to sleep onset. During the afternoon observations these children were sleeping less and spent more time awake, active and alert, which may have explained their lesser difficulties getting to sleep at night. They could have had a greater need

Table 3.4 Bedtime behaviors for massage therapy and reading control group for the first vs last day of study

	Massage		Control	
	First day	Last day	First day	Last day
Child behaviors				
No. disruptive behaviors	3.1	1.7[a]	3.3	2.8
Bedtime preparation (min.)	45.0	32.1	47.5	40.1[a]
Sleep onset latency (min.)	43.3	25.6[a]	45.7	45.0
Parent response to child				
Difficulty putting child to sleep	1.8	3.3[a]	2.1	2.4
Parental anxiety	2.2	3.8[a]	2.2	3.0
Child's activity level	1.6	3.8	1.8	2.7
Improvement in behavior	3.5	2.7[a]	3.5	3.0
Ease in falling asleep (%)	100.0	33.0[a]	100.0	70.0

[a]Significant differences between columns.

Table 3.5 Sleep observation measures on the first and last days of the study for the massage and control group

	Massage		Control	
Behavior observations	First day	Last day	First day	Last day
Deep sleep	17.8	0.0[a]	21.3	48.0
Active sleep	30.3	0.0[a]	28.4	43.6
Drowsy	11.9	1.6	8.6	1.5
Alert inactive	6.6	24.3[a]	6.0	1.9
Alert active	20.9	59.6[a]	20.0	1.2
Fussing	1.9	4.0	1.0	1.0
Multiple limb movements	44.9	66.9[a]	44.7	22.2
Mouthing	1.5	0.0[a]	1.6	2.3
Smiling	1.9	5.8[a]	1.0	1.0

[a]Significant differences between columns.

for sleep at night, as evidenced by the fewer number of disruptive behaviors and the shorter latency to sleep at night. In addition, finding it less difficult to get their children to sleep probably contributed to the parents feeling less anxiety by the end of the study.

Although the underlying mechanism is not clear, massage therapy has also contributed to alert, wakeful activity in adults (Field et al 1996). In this study EEG waves changed in the direction of heightened alertness following massage therapy sessions, and greater alertness translated into improved performance on mathematical problems (less time required and greater accuracy).

In addition to reducing activity or arousal levels, it is also possible that the physical contact of massage therapy reduced stress hormones, as has been noted in other studies on infants (Field et al 1996). Unfortunately, stress hormones were not measured in this study, but these data combined suggest that additional physical contact with the parent at bedtime may reduce stress. If this is true, the goal of previous behavioral interventions to help infants sleep without disturbing their parents may be at odds with the infant's biological needs. The group differences in this study might have also been exaggerated by the reading group having less physical contact than usual at bedtime. Future studies might benefit from monitoring stress hormones and activity levels more objectively, for example, by the time-lapse video or motility mattress monitors during nighttime sleep rather than depending on the potentially more biased parent reports. Studies could also be conducted on sleep patterns in cultures that routinely massage their infants, such as the East Indian culture. In the interim, these results suggest that massage therapy may be a cost-effective treatment for reducing sleep problems in infants and toddlers.

References

Brazelton TB 1973 Neonatal Behavior Assessment Scale. Spastics International Medical Publications, London.

Diego M, Field T, Sanders C, et al 2003 Massage therapy of moderate and light pressure and vibrator effects on EEG and heart rate. International Journal of Neuroscience 114:31–44.

Dieter J, Field T, Hernandez-Reif M, et al 2003 Stable preterm infants gain more weight and sleep less after five days of massage therapy. Journal of Pediatrics and Psychology 28(6):403–411.

Ferber R 1985 Behavioral 'insomnia' in the child. Psychological Clinics of North America 10:641–653.

Ferber SG, Kuint J, Weller A, et al 2002 Massage therapy by mothers and trained professionals enhances weight gain in preterm infants. Early Human Development 67:37–45.

Field T 1988 Stimulation of preterm infants. Pediatrics in Review 10:149–154.

Field T 2001 Massage therapy facilitates weight gain in preterm infants. Directions in Psychological Science 10(2):51–54.

Field T, Hernandez-Reif M 2001 Sleep problems in infants decrease following massage therapy. Early Child Development and Care 168:95–104.

Field T, Schanberg SM, Scafidi F, et al 1986 Tactile/kinesthetic stimulation effects on preterm neonates. Pediatrics 77:654–658.

Field T, Scafidi F, Schanberg SM 1987 Massage of preterm newborns to improve growth and development. Pediatric Nursing 13:385–387.

Field T, Morrow C, Valdeon C, et al 1992 Massage therapy reduces anxiety in child and adolescent psychiatric patients. Journal of the American Academy of Child and Adolescent Psychiatry 31:125–131.

Field T, Grizzle N, Scafidi F, et al 1996 Massage therapy for infants of depressed mothers. Infant Behavior and Development 19:107–112.

Field T, Hernandez-Reif M, Diego M, et al 2004 Massage therapy by parents improves early growth and development. Infant Behavior and Development 27(4):435–442.

Guthertz M, Field T 1989 Lap computer or on-line coding and data analysis for laboratory and field observations. Infant Behavior and Development 12:305–319.

Jinon S 1996 The effect of infant massage on growth of the preterm infant. In: Yarbes-Almirante C, De Luma M (eds) Increasing sage and successful pregnancy. Elsevier Science, Amsterdam, pp 265–269.

Kuhn C, Schanberg S, Field T, et al 1991 Tactile-kinesthetic stimulation effects on sympathetic and adrenocortical function in preterm infants. Journal of Pediatrics 119:434–440.

Lester B, Als H, Brazelton T B 1982 Regional obstetric anesthesia and newborn behavior: a reanalysis toward synergistic effects. Child Development 53:687–692.

McClure V 1989 Infant massage: a handbook for loving parents. Bantam Books, New York.

McKechnie A, Wilson F, Watson N, et al 1983 Anxiety states: a preliminary report on the value of connective tissue massage. Journal of Psychosomatic Research 27:125–129.

Moyer-Mileur L, Luetkemeier M, Boomer L, et al 1995 Effect of physical activity on bone mineralization in premature infants. Journal of Pediatrics 127:620–625.

Ottenbacher KJ, Muller L, Brandt D, et al 1987 The effectiveness of tactile stimulation as a form of early intervention: a quantitative evaluation. Journal of Developmental and Behavioral Pediatrics 8:68–76.

Pauk J, Kuhn C, Field T, 1986 Positive effects of tactile versus kinesthetic or vestibular stimulation on neuroendocrine and ODC activity in maternally deprived rat pups. Life Science 39(22):2081–2087.

Salzarulo P, Chevalier A 1983 Sleep problems in children and their relationship with early disturbances of the waking-sleeping rhythms. Sleep 6:47–51.

Scafidi F, Field T, Schanberg SM, et al 1986 Effects of tactile/kinesthetic stimulation on the clinical course and sleep/wake behavior of preterm neonates. Infant Behavior and Development 9:91–105.

Scafidi F, Field T, Schanberg SM, et al 1990 Massage stimulation growth in preterm infants: a replication. Infant Behavior and Development 13:167–188.

Schanberg S, Field T 1987 Sensory deprivation stress and supplemental stimulation in the rat pup and preterm human neonate. Child Development 58(6):1431–1447.

Shoemaker JK, Tiidus PM, Mader R 1997 Failure of manual massage to alter limb blood flow: measures by Doppler ultrasound. Medicine and Science in Sports and Exercise 29:610–614.

Sullivan SJ, Williams LR, Seaborne DE, et al 1991 Effects of massage on alpha motorneuron excitability. Physical Therapy 71:555–560.

Thoman E 1975 Early development of sleeping behavior in infants. In: Ellis N (ed.) Aberrant development in infancy. Erlbaum, Hillsdale, NJ, pp 132–138.

Uvnas-Moberg K, Widstrom A, Marchini G, et al 1987 Release of GI hormones in mother and infant by sensory stimulation. Acta Paediatrica Scandinavica 76:851–860.

Wheeden A, Scafidi F, Field T, et al 1993 Massage effects on cocaine-exposed preterm neonates. Journal of Developmental and Behavioral Pediatrics 14:318–322.

Chapter **4**

Increasing attentiveness

CHAPTER CONTENTS

The vagus nerve may be responsible for mediating the effects of massage therapy on attentiveness. In many studies, vagal activity has been shown to increase and heart rate to decrease. Increased attentiveness is typically associated with decreased heart rate. The vagus has a branch to the heart and effectively slows heart rate. A particular pattern of electroencephalogram (EEG) is also associated with enhanced attentiveness. This pattern is usually an elevation of alpha, beta and theta activity, and a decrease in delta activity. In the following studies, attentiveness and related performance were studied in infants, preschoolers, school-age children, adolescents, and adults.

In the first study, infants who received a brief period of massage before a visual attention task were noted to show more visual attentiveness on the task and to habituate or learn stimulus properties faster than those who did not receive massage (Cigales et al 1997). In a study on preschool-age children, the preschoolers were massaged briefly before taking an IQ test (Hart et al 1998). Those preschoolers who received the brief massage were noted to perform better, particularly on the blocks and pegs tasks of the IQ test. In the third study, children with autism were provided with massage therapy every night before bedtime, and they were noted not only to have better sleep patterns but also to show more on-task behavior in the classrooms (Escalona et al 2001). In a similar study on adolescents with attention disorder, massages led to less hyperactive behavior and more on-task performance in the classroom (Field et al 1998). In studies assessing the EEG patterns associated with massage therapy, moderate-pressure massage vs light massage was associated with enhanced attentiveness, including slower heart rate, and EEG patterns associated with enhanced attentiveness (Diego et al 2004). Similarly, in a study on aroma and EEG patterns, the lavender aroma was associated with increased relaxation and attentiveness as measured by behavior and EEG activity (Diego et al 1998).

STUDY 1: MASSAGE ENHANCES COGNITIVE PERFORMANCE IN NORMAL INFANTS

Massage helps performance on the habituation cluster of the Brazelton Scale (Scafidi et al 1990). In the typical habituation procedure, the infant's baseline duration of looking at a stimulus is established. The stimulus is then presented repeatedly until the visual fixation response reaches a habituation criterion, for example, visual fixation durations of 50% or less of baseline on two consecutive trials. Test trials are then presented, in which some aspect of the stimulus is changed, and response recovery (i.e. dishabituation) is assessed. An increase in the infant's visual fixation duration above his or her habituation level indicates that the infant has discriminated the changed stimulus. It should be possible to enhance infants' response habituation rate and/or recovery by facilitating optimal arousal before and during habituation.

A study conducted on the effects of massage on infants' performance on an audiovisual habituation task (Cigales et al 1997) involved a brief massage given prior to the task. Although this had not yet been done with infants, research on adults suggested that brain waves (EEG alpha, beta and delta) changed in the direction of heightened alertness following massage, and, in turn, adults performed math computations faster and with fewer errors (Field et al 1997a).

Method

Participants and procedure

Fifty-six 4-month-old infants were randomly assigned to either a 'massage' condition or 'play' condition. Infants in the 'massage' condition were given

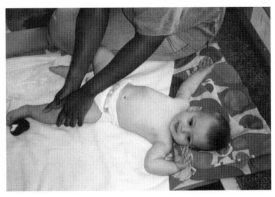

Figure 4.1   Infant massage in cognitive performance test.

an 8-minute massage (Fig. 4.1). The massage consisted of deep, but gentle, rubbing and stroking of the chest, legs, feet, arms, and hands. The infants were then turned over onto their stomachs to massage their neck, head, and back. Infants in the play group did not receive massage, but were entertained with a red teething ring for 8 minutes.

For the habituation procedure, the infants were seated in an infant seat facing the video monitor approximately 16 in. (40.64 cm) away. The stimuli were presented on the video monitor one at a time on sequential trials. The habituation stimulus films consisted of two toy hammers. One hammer was red and was depicted against a black background, and the other was blue against a gray background. Both hammers were depicted tapping out the same rhythm, but one tapped at a slow tempo and the other tapped at a comparatively fast tempo.

An observer recorded the onset and offset on the infant's looking at the stimulus. A laptop computer was used to record the duration of looking at each stimulus. The looking durations were averaged across the first two habituation trials to obtain a baseline of the infant's attention to the stimuli. The stimuli were alternated across trials until the infant met the habituation criterion. To meet the criterion, the infant's looking durations had to decrease to 50% or less of the baseline level on two consecutive trials. Once the habituation criterion was met, the infant was presented two post-habituation trials, which consisted of continued presentations of the habituation stimuli.

Two test (dishabituation) trials were immediately presented following the post-habituation trials. In the test trials the opposite color–tempo stimulus was presented. For example, if the habituation stimuli had been red–fast, blue–slow, the test trials consisted of red–slow, blue–fast. If infants could discriminate the change in color–tempo relations, their looking time was expected to increase to above post-habituation levels. Finally, a control trial (C2) was presented consisting of the control stimulus shown during C1.

Table 4.1 Means for massage and play conditions

	Massage	Play
Post–habituation	6.9	6.8
Test trials (ms)	20.1[a]	12.6[b]

[a,b]Means with different superscripts differ significantly from each other.

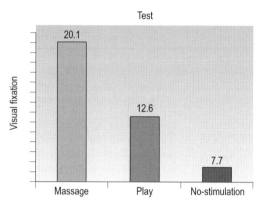

Figure 4.2 Massaged infants looked significantly longer on the test trials than the play group.

Results

The data analyses revealed that the massage group looked significantly longer in the test trials than on the post-habituation trials, whereas the play group did not (see Table 4.1; Fig. 4.2). These findings suggest that only infants who received massage discriminated the test stimuli from the habituation stimuli.

Discussion

The results indicated that massage had beneficial effects on infants' discrimination of different color–tempo stimuli. Lecuyer (1989) suggested that response habituation and recovery may reflect infants' control of attentional processes. Thus, massaged infants may have attended to the object–tempo relations, whereas infants in the other group may have attended to the global aspects of the stimuli. Whether massage results in improved attentional or memory processes, or both, remains to be determined, as well as the long-term implications of massage therapy on cognitive development.

Although the present findings suggest that massage can enhance infants' cognitive performance, such effects may be only transient. Future research should also investigate the potential remedial effects of massage among developmentally delayed or at-risk infants.

STUDY 2: PRESCHOOLERS' COGNITIVE PERFORMANCE IMPROVES FOLLOWING MASSAGE

Massage therapy enhances cognitive functioning. Adults who received a chair massage in their office showed increased speed and accuracy on math computations, along with EEG wave changes suggesting heightened alertness (Field et al 1996a). In another study on the cognitive performance of infants, those who received a massage prior to an audiovisual task showed greater response recovery following habituation, again suggesting superior cognitive performance (Cigales et al 1997). The present study assessed massage effects on the cognitive performance of preschoolers.

Method

Participants and procedure

Twenty preschoolers were seen individually in their classroom by a graduate student experimenter who was 'blind' to the study's hypotheses. After becoming acquainted with the experimenter, each child was tested on the cognitive performance tasks (Wechsler Preschool and Primary Scale of Intelligence—Revised [WPPSI-R]; Wechsler 1989). Immediately following the pre-test session, children in the massage therapy group received a 15-minute massage from a massage therapist and children in the play control group spent 15 minutes reading stories with an experimenter. Afterward, the children were tested in the post-test session by the experimenter.

Wechsler Preschool and Primary Scale of Intelligence—Revised (WPPSI-R)
(Wechsler 1989)
Three perceptual-motor (performance) subtests were administered:

1. Block Design, requiring the child to analyze and reproduce patterns made from two-colored blocks.
2. Animal Pegs, requiring the child to place pegs of the correct colors in holes.
3. Mazes, in which the child was required to solve pencil-and-paper mazes.

Massage therapy A massage therapist gave the children in the massage therapy group a 15-minute massage, comprising two standardized phases. In the first phase, the child was placed in a supine position and stroked in the following sequence: (1) face: (a) strokes along both sides of the face, (b) flats of fingers across the forehead, (c) circular strokes over the temples and the hinge of the jaw, and (d) flat fingers strokes over the nose, cheeks, jaw, and chin; (2) stomach: (a) hand-over-hand strokes in a paddlewheel fashion, avoiding the ribs and the tip of the rib cage, (b) circular motion with fingers in a clockwise direction starting at the appendix; (3) legs: (a) strokes from hip to foot, (b) squeezing and twisting in a wringing motion from hip to foot, (c) massaging the foot and toes, (d) stretching the Achilles tendon, and (e) stroking the legs upward toward the heart; (4) arms: (a) strokes from the shoulders to the hands, using (b) same procedure as for the legs.

For the second phase, with the subject in a prone position, the child was massaged in the following sequence: (1) downward strokes along the back, (2) hand-over-hand movements from the upper back to the hip, (3) hands from side to side across the back, including the sides, (4) circular motion from head to hips along, but not touching the spine, (5) simultaneous strokes over the sides of the back from the middle to the sides, (6) rubbing and kneading shoulder muscles, (7) rubbing the neck, (8) strokes along the length of the back, and (9) strokes from crown to feet.

Play Children in the play control group spent 15 minutes with the experimenter reading a Dr Seuss story. The child and experimenter were seated close together on a carpeted area for this session.

Results

As can be seen in Table 4.2, performance on Block Design improved following massage therapy but not following play. Accuracy on Animal Pegs remained stable following massage therapy, but deteriorated following play.

Discussion

Massage therapy enhanced the cognitive performance of these preschoolers, consistent with similar studies on infants and adults (Cigales et al 1997, Field et al 1996a). The group differences may have related to the massaged children becoming increasingly alert following the massage, not unlike the heightened alertness shown by wave changes in adults following massage. EEG might be measured in a future study of this kind with preschoolers.

That preschoolers' cognitive performance is enhanced by massage therapy raises some concern, since little touch takes place in preschools and progressively less positive touch occurs across ages from the infant to toddler to preschool nurseries (Field et al 1994). Since the long-term effects of massage therapy have not yet been established, further studies are needed to determine the extent to which touch therapy needs to be incorporated in the preschool curriculum.

Table 4.2 Mean WPPSI subtest scores

	Massage		Play	
	Pre-	Post-	Pre-	Post-
Blocks	11.3[a]	13.1[b]	11.0[a]	11.3[a]
Animal pegs: accuracy	19.3[a]	19.7[a]	19.6[a]	17.4[b]

[a,b]Means bearing different superscripts differ.

STUDY 3: AUTISM SYMPTOMS DECREASE FOLLOWING MASSAGE THERAPY

Several traditional and non-traditional treatments for children with autism have been researched, but no single treatment modality has been effective (Tsai 1992). Medications have improved some symptoms (Mesibov et al 1997). Imitation by parents has been effective (Dawson & Galpert 1990), as has behavior modification in highly structured environments (Rogers 1999, Tsai 1992). Massage therapy has been effective for children with autism in at least one study. In that study, Field and colleagues (Field et al 1997b) reported positive effects following 1 month of massage therapy conducted twice weekly for 20 minutes by massage therapists. These effects included less touch aversion and fewer autistic behaviors such as orienting to sounds and stereotypic behaviors, and more on-task behavior and social relatedness during classroom behavior observations.

The present study was designed to have parents administer the massage therapy so that the children could receive the treatment on a daily basis at no cost (Escalona et al 2001). Having daily massages before bedtime was expected to help reduce sleep problems frequently noted in these children (Klinger & Dawson 1996), just as it had in previous studies on preschool children with sleep problems (Field et al 1996a, Klinger & Dawson 1996) and depressed children who had fewer nightwakings following a week of daily massages (Field et al 1992). The present study followed the same massage therapy and assessment procedures as the Field et al (1997b) study, except that the children's parents were trained by massage therapists to administer the massages on a daily basis before the children's bedtime instead of therapists massaging the children twice weekly during class time. More frequent massages by a familiar person (the parent) were expected to yield greater improvement in the child's sleep and preschool behaviors.

Method

Participants

Twenty children with autism ranging in age from 3 to 6 years were recruited from a school for children with autism. The children were randomly assigned from the same developmental level classrooms to massage therapy and reading attention control groups. We administered the Preschool Performance Scale (Schopler & Reichler 1979) and found that the two groups did not differ in their scores. The parents in both groups were told that 'reading stories and massaging might increase relaxation and sleep in their children'.

Procedure

Massage therapy group   The children in this group received parent (mostly mothers) massage therapy for 15 minutes just prior to bedtime every day for a month. Parents were trained by a massage therapist in the same massage procedure used in our previous study (Field et al 1997b). This involved firmly massaging with moderate pressure five regions of the child's body in the following sequence: arms and hands, legs, front, and back.

Attention control group   The parents of the children in the attention control group were asked to read a Dr Seuss story to their children for 15 minutes just prior to bedtime every night for a month. After the completion of the study the parents in the control group also received instructions in massage therapy.

Assessments

The children in both groups were assessed on the first and last days of the study using the same measures used by Field et al (1997b) in order to have comparative data, including the revised Conners Teacher and Parent Scales (Conners 1997), classroom and playground behavior observations, and sleep diaries.

Revised Conners Scales   The revised Conners Scales (Conners 1997) on children's behaviors were completed by the children's teacher (who was blind to the group assignment of the children) and parents (the primary caregiver) on the first and last days of the study.

Classroom and playground behavior observations   Behavior observations were conducted in the classroom and on the playground on the first and last days of the month-long study. Research associates, who were blind to the children's group assignment, recorded these behaviors on time sample unit sheets every 10 seconds for a total of 15 minutes per child. The behaviors were taken from the Field et al (1997b) study and included positive response to touch, on-task behavior, stereotypical behavior, and social relatedness to the teacher.

Sleep diaries   Parents also recorded their children's sleep behavior in sleep diaries on the first night and on the night before the last day of the study. These diaries included the amount of fussing, restlessness, crying, self-stimulating behavior, and the number of times the children left the bed. These behaviors were rated on 5-point Likert Scales (1 = not at all, 2 = a little, 3 = fair amount, 4 = a lot, 5 = extreme). This scale was designed for the current study.

Results

Greater improvement was noted for the massage therapy group from the first to the last day on the teachers' ratings for the Emotional index (62 to 55 vs 62 to 60), and the DSM-IV (inattentiveness; 62 to 51 vs 60 to 62). The parents' ratings also indicated improvement for the massage therapy group on the Attention-deficit/hyperactivity disorder (ADHD) index (66 to 60 vs 65 to 64), restless impulsive behavior (66 to 60 vs 66 to 63), the Emotional index (58 to 54 vs 55 to 55), and the DSM-IV (inattentiveness; 62 to 56 vs 63 to 61).

Classroom observations indicated a greater decrease in stereotypical behaviors (8% to <1% vs 5% to 2%) and a greater increase in on-task behavior (81% to 94% vs 81% to 91%) from the first to the last day for the massage group. Playground observations indicated a greater decrease from the first to the last day of the study in the frequency of stereotypical behaviors (13% to 2% vs 12% to 8%), and a greater increase in social relatedness toward the teacher (14% to 20% vs 14% to 11%) in the massage therapy group. Change scores for sleep behaviors indicated greater declines for the massage therapy group on the following behaviors: fussing/ restlessness, crying, self-stimulating behavior, and getting out of bed.

Discussion

The clinical significance of this study is that two problems that impair the classroom performance of children with autism, namely off-task behavior (Fig. 4.3A) and sleep problems (Fig. 4.3B), were improved. This increased attentiveness is similar to the increased on-task behavior noted in the earlier massage therapy study by Field and colleagues (Field et al 1997b). Although the underlying mechanism for this enhanced attentiveness is not known, massage therapy has also been noted to enhance vagal activity (Field 1998), which is highly correlated with attentiveness (Porges 1997). Stereotypical behaviors also decreased in the classroom and on the playground, again consistent with the decrease in stereotypical behaviors in our earlier massage therapy study (Field et al 1997b).

The behavior changes could have related to the children being more rested from having slept better, as reflected in their lower levels of fussing, crying,

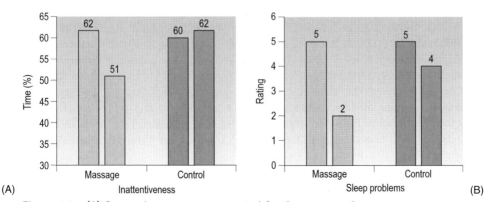

Figure 4.3 (A) Greater improvement was noted for the massage therapy group compared to controls on attentiveness. (B) Sleep problems improved in children with autism following massage therapy.

self-stimulating and getting-out-of-bed behaviors. However, the sleep ratings may have been biased because the parents were not blind to their child's group assignment. In addition, the parents expressed 'really liking' the massage, suggesting the possibility of a Hawthorne effect (i.e. showing improvement related to enjoyment). Improved sleep may derive from the increase in vagal activity typically noted following massage therapy. A future study would desirably monitor sleep with the more objective activity meters (Eaton et al 1988). Other measures such as vagal activity and stress hormone assays might also better inform us regarding potential underlying mechanisms.

STUDY 4: MASSAGE THERAPY IMPROVES MOOD AND BEHAVIOR OF STUDENTS WITH ATTENTION–DEFICIT/HYPERACTIVITY DISORDER

ADHD is the most recent diagnostic label for children and adolescents who present with attention, impulse control, and overactivity problems. At least 10% of behavior problems seen in general pediatric settings are due to ADHD, and up to 50% in some child and adolescent psychiatric samples. Children with ADHD may vary considerably in their symptoms. However, they are often described as having chronic difficulties in regard to inattention, impulsivity, and overactivity.

Numerous studies (double-blind, placebo-controlled) have concluded that stimulants are more effective in ameliorating ADHD's core behavioral symptoms of hyperactivity, impulsivity, and inattentiveness than placebos, non-pharmacological therapies, or no treatment (Spencer et al 2002). This mode of treatment continues to be controversial in this population because of its behavior-modifying properties and associated side-effects. A combined intervention of medication management and behavioral treatment has been found to be more successful than either approach alone in reducing core ADHD symptoms in children (Rieppi et al 2002).

A non-medication intervention that has only recently been explored in children with ADHD is massage therapy. In a recent study, adolescents with ADHD who received 10 massage treatments over the course of 2 weeks rated themselves as happier than those who participated in relaxation therapy. Observers rated the massage therapy group as less fidgety, and teachers reported more on-task behavior, when compared to the relaxation therapy group (Field et al 1998). Teachers also noticed a significant decrease in hyperactivity for the massage therapy group but not for the relaxation therapy group.

The underlying mechanism by which massage therapy decreases hyperactivity and increases attentiveness is not clear, although physiological and biochemical data from the Field et al (1996a, 1998) studies suggest some possibilities, including that brain waves are altered in the direction of heightened alertness (see Field et al 1996a). In addition, increased vagal tone (and thus increased parasympathetic activity) has been noted during massage therapy, and this increase is often associated with enhanced attentiveness and a more relaxed state (Porges 1991). Massage therapy may enhance vagal control of the heart by improving a deficient physiological inhibitory system. This, in turn, might help hyperactive or learning-disordered children to mediate and inhibit spontaneous activity, and thereby increase their level of attentiveness.

In the present investigation (Khilnani et al 2003), massage therapy was selected as an additional treatment for those receiving ongoing intervention, because prior studies found that it exceeded the effects of relaxation therapy and other stress-management treatments used in various clinical samples, including youths with ADHD (Field et al 1992, 1998). Previous massage studies also reported increases in vagal tone during massage therapy (Field 1995). It would follow that massage therapy might improve attention in those with ADHD by promoting vagal control of heart rate.

The following hypotheses were tested:

1. Students in the massage therapy group would rate themselves as happier and feeling better post-massage on both assessment days when compared to those in the wait-list control group.
2. The massage therapy group would show a significant reduction in behavioral problems in the classroom, specifically hyperactivity and inattention (based on teacher ratings).
3. The massage therapy group would show a significant decrease in depressed mood.

Method

Participants

Parental consent forms were distributed to all students attending a learning center for children and adolescents with academic and behavioral problems. The sample consisted of the first 30 students who returned signed consent forms and who had a current DSM-IV diagnosis of ADHD. The participants were between the ages of 7 and 18 years (mean = 13 years).

Procedure

Massage therapy The students were randomly assigned to a massage therapy group or wait-list control group. The massages were held in a large, quiet, room located in the school building. Each student in the massage therapy group received two 20-minute massages per week for a total of nine treatment sessions. Massages were conducted on portable massage tables, and all participants remained fully clothed during each massage. Students were told that the massages might help them relax. The massage entailed moderate-pressure stroking for 4-minute periods in each of five regions: head/neck, arms, torso, legs, and back. Massage while in the supine position lasted 10 minutes and included lateral stroking of the forehead, gentle rocking (torso and legs), and continuous stretching of the Achilles tendon. Massage while in the prone position also lasted 10 minutes and included lateral lumbar stretches, neck squeezes, and kneading of the back. Last-day assessments were conducted after the eighth (penultimate) massage session instead of the ninth, in order to minimize potential termination effects such as feeling disappointed that the massages were over.

Wait–list control group   Participants in this group were informed that they would have an opportunity to experience the massage procedure on a voluntary basis during the following month.

Short-term measures

Mood state   Information about mood state was collected through the developmentally appropriate use of pictorial self-reports. A faces scale was used to provide an estimate of the participant's experiences. Drawings of four faces ranging from sad (scored as 1) to happy (scored as 4) were presented to the participants before and after the first and last assessment sessions. A drawing of a thermometer with a vertical scale was used as a second measure of mood state, ranging from zero (i.e. 'not feeling good at all') to 10 (i.e. 'best I have ever felt'), that best described the way they felt.

Long-term measures

Teachers (who were blind to group assignment) were asked to complete the Conners Teacher Rating Scale, which is one of the most widely-used behavior rating scales for assessing hyperactivity, conduct problems, emotional–indulgent, anxious–passive, asocial, and daydream/attention problems.

Immediate effects   On the faces scale, the massage therapy group reported feeling happier after the first- and last-day sessions (see Table 4.3). On the thermometer scale, the massage therapy group rated themselves as feeling better after the first- and last-day sessions.

Longer–term effect   There were significant effects showing reductions in hyperactivity and daydreaming/inattention only for the massage therapy group (See Table 4.3).

Discussion

The present findings are consistent with a recent massage therapy study in which adolescents with ADHD showed improvements in fidgetiness, hyperactivity, on-task behavior (Fig. 4.4), and subjective feelings of happiness (Field et al 1998), and another study that reported less anxiety after massage therapy (Shulman & Jones 1996). The enhanced mood states found in the present study may have contributed to the improved classroom behavior. Teacher ratings of students with ADHD who participated in the massage therapy

Table 4.3   Means for massage versus control group pre-/post-session and first and last day measures

	Massage group				Control group			
	First day		Last day		First day		Last day	
Variables	Pre-	Post-	Pre-	Post-	Pre-	Post-	Pre-	Post-
Mood/stress								
Faces	3.1[a]	3.5[b]	3.3[a]	3.7[b]	3.3[a]	3.4[a]	3.7[a]	3.7[a]
Thermometer	6.3[a]	7.8[b]	6.9[a]	8.7[b]	7.5[a]	7.8[a]	8.4[a]	8.6[a]
Behavior (T scores)	First day		Last day		First day		Last day	
Hyperactivity	62.9[a]		54.2[b]		63.0[a]		60.5[a]	
Conduct problems	58.7[a]		54.1[a]		57.4[a]		57.0[a]	
Emotional–indulgent	63.9[a]		55.3[b]		65.9[a]		61.5[b]	
Anxious–passive	48.9[a]		44.3[b]		53.5[a]		56.0[a]	
Asocial	47.8[a]		46.7[a]		54.5[a]		55.3[a]	
Daydreams	61.2[a]		52.7[b]		58.2[a]		56.4[a]	

[a,b]Different letter superscripts indicate significant differences within groups using post-hoc comparison t-tests.

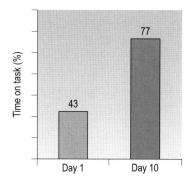

Figure 4.4   On-task behavior improved in children and adolescents with ADHD following massage therapy.

suggest that the therapy reduced the problems most associated with ADHD, namely hyperactivity and daydreaming/inattention, over the course of the treatment period. The convergence of self-report measures and teacher ratings highlights both the immediate and longer-term effectiveness of massage therapy and supports the use of this treatment with this population.

Future studies are needed to ascertain how massage therapy impacts on academic achievement in students with ADHD. Incorporating additional measures such as vagal tone and EEG might also help explain the relationship between massage therapy and on-task behavior in children and adolescents with ADHD. Several studies suggest that massage therapy enhances cognitive performance (Hart et al 1998), including improved math computations following massage therapy and EEG changes suggesting a pattern of heightened alertness (Field et al 1996a). In the Hart et al (1998) study massaged children improved on their performance on Block Design and Animal Pegs subtests of the WPPSI-R. The increased attentiveness observed in classroom behavior using the Conners Scale in the present study could be related to enhanced vagal activity that occurs during massage therapy (Field 1990). Increased cardiac vagal control via the parasympathetic nervous system may enhance the ability of the hyperactive child to mediate spontaneous activity (Porges 1998).

Although massage therapy appears to effectively improve the short-term mood state in students with ADHD and decrease their problem behaviors in the classroom, its efficacy needs to be compared to other treatments such as stimulant medications and other complementary therapies such as Tai Chi, a therapy that has also been shown to be effective in children with ADHD (Hernandez-Reif et al 1999). In addition, the present study could not, of course, be a double-blind study as the participants were inevitably aware that they were receiving massage therapy. Assessing whether the massage therapy effects generalized to other settings in addition to the classroom would have also been an important outcome to explore. For example, parent reports on the behavior of their children/adolescents (e.g. Conners Parent Rating Scale) could be employed in future studies to document the effects of massage therapy noticed in the home. Nonetheless, teacher ratings concurred with self-reports, suggesting that massage therapy could become an important treatment in the multimodal management of ADHD.

STUDY 5: MASSAGE THERAPY OF MODERATE AND LIGHT PRESSURE AND VIBRATOR EFFECTS ON EEG AND HEART RATE

Few controlled studies have evaluated the different pressure or different massage therapy techniques. One study that assessed blood flow in response to deep-pressure stroking versus percussion movements revealed that only the percussion movements increased blood flow (Hovind & Nielsen 1974). In another study assessing alpha motor neuron excitability, deep-pressure massage reduced H-reflex excitability, whereas light fingertip pressure did not (Sullivan et al 1991). This finding supports data from other studies that have shown that deep-pressure stroking produces significant physiological and psychological effects, whereas light-pressure stroking does not. For example, one study assessing limb blood flow by Doppler ultrasound failed to show any effects with light-pressure stroking (Shoemaker et al 1997). In contrast, a study assessing the effects of deep-pressure massage found increased range of motion and changes in electroneuromyograpy (ENMG) following treatment (McKechnie et al 1983). In this pilot study, mean heart rate (BPM) and ENMG activity decreased while skin resistance (SRL) increased in response to connective tissue massage (deep pressure). Vibratory stimulation has been shown to enhance relaxation and decrease pain in adults (Lundeberg et al 1984, Ottoson et al 1981).

The present study assessed the physiological and psychological effects of three different massage therapy techniques, including light-pressure and deep-pressure massage provided by hands and vibratory stimulation provided by a mechanical massager (Thumper Mini Pro, Model # NAOOP, Worldwide Patents) (Diego et al 2004). The physiological effects of the three massage conditions were assessed by monitoring heart rate and EEG data from each participant and assessing anxiety and stress on self-report scales.

As in previous studies, moderate-pressure stimulation was expected to decrease heart rate, negative affect and anxiety. EEG for this condition was expected to reflect increased delta and decreased alpha and beta power, suggesting a pattern of relaxation and alertness and a shift toward greater left-frontal EEG asymmetry, suggesting greater positive affect. No specific effects were hypothesized for the low-pressure or the vibratory stimulation groups.

Method

Participants

The sample included 36 faculty and staff members of a large urban medical school. The participants were randomly assigned to a light-pressure touch, moderate-pressure touch, or vibratory stimulation condition. Demographics are shown in Table 4.4.

Table 4.4   Means (and standard deviations) for demographics of light- and moderate-pressure massage and vibratory stimulation groups

	Light (N = 12)	Moderate (N = 12)	Vibratory (N = 12)	
Age	29.92	29.58	27.42	$F(2, 33) = 0.25$, NS[a]
	(10.29)	(8.32)	(9.57)	
SES	2.25	2.75	2.75	$F(2, 33) = 2.59$, NS
	(0.62)	(0.75)	(0.45)	
Gender				
Male	58%	17%	50%	$X^2 (2) = 4.80$, $p =$ NS
Female	42%	83%	50%	
Ethnicity				$X^2 (6) = 6.00$, $p =$ NS
Caucasian	33%	67%	75%	
African-American	8%	8%	8%	
Hispanic	42%	17%	17%	
Other	17%	8%	0%	
Touch aversion	35.08	34.25	35.75	$F(2, 33) = 0.27$, NS
	(5.59)	(3.82)	(5.56)	

[a]NS: not significant.

Assessment procedure

The procedure was conducted in the following order: (1) an EEG cap was positioned on the participant's head, (2) EKG electrodes were placed along the participant's arms, (3) participants completed the session baseline measures, including the demographic questionnaire, the State Anxiety Inventory (STAI; Spielberger et al 1970), the visual analog stress/relaxation scale, and the Touch Aversion Questionnaire, (4) a 3-minute baseline followed by the 10-minute massage was given and a 3-minute post-session during which EEG and EKG were continuously recorded, followed by (6) the STAI and the visual analog stress/relaxation scale.

EEG and EKG procedures

EEG was recorded for 3-minute periods prior to, 10-minutes during, and 3-minutes after the massage, with the subject's eyes closed. The EEG was recorded using a lycra stretchable cap (Electro-Cap, Inc., OH, USA) positioned on the participant's head. EKG was obtained for 3 minutes pre-, during, and post-massage by placing three EKG electrodes in a standard configuration along the participant's inner arms.

Touch Aversion Questionnaire

The Touch Aversion Questionnaire is a 24-item questionnaire which measures sensitivity to touch, with 1 = 'no', 2 = 'a little' and 3 = 'a lot'. Characteristic items include 'Do fuzzy shirts bother you?' and 'Does it bother you to have your face touched?'

Pre-/post-self-report measures

The following measures were used to assess the immediate effects of the different types of massage. The STAI (Spielberger et al 1970) is a 20-item scale which measures transitory anxiety levels in terms of severity, with 1 = 'not so much' and 4 = 'very much'. Characteristic items include 'I feel tense' and 'I feel relaxed'. A visual analog scale was used to assess the stressed/relaxed state with a score of 0 = 'very tense' and a score of 10 = 'very relaxed'.

Massage procedure

Following a 3-minute baseline recording, participants received a moderate-pressure massage, a light-pressure massage or a vibratory massage. Participants in all conditions received 10 minutes of stimulation to the back, shoulders and arms by a trained massage therapist, while sitting fully clothed in a standard massage chair. The moderate-pressure massage consisted of long, deep-pressure stroking and squeezing; the light-pressure massage consisted of long, light-pressure stroking, and the vibratory massage consisted of the Thumper (hand-held massager) vibrating at 40Hz on the deep pressure setting.

The massage therapists were trained on the protocol and did not play another role in the study. All therapists were kept blind to the pressure hypothesis. Intermittent re-evaluation by the researchers ensured protocol compliance, especially with respect to the amount of pressure provided. Those therapists providing the light-pressure massage did not perform deep-pressure massage or vibratory massage and vice versa.

Results

Participants in the moderate massage group reported a greater decrease in self-reported stress than participants in the light massage or the vibratory massage group. A trend for the light massage suggested a decrease in frontal delta power during and following light massage. A trend for the moderate massage group suggested an increase in frontal delta power during the moderate-pressure massage procedure (see Table 4.5). Moderate-pressure massage resulted in the greatest proportion of adults exhibiting a shift towards left frontal EEG asymmetry (90% vs 75% for the light-pressure massage and 56% for the vibratory stimulation). Only the moderate-pressure massage group exhibited a trend towards left frontal EEG asymmetry.

The moderate-pressure massage group showed a decrease in heart rate during the massage, which continued into the post-session, and the light massage group showed a significant increase in heart rate following the massage. The vibratory stimulation group also exhibited an increase in heart rate following the massage (Fig. 4.5).

Table 4.5 Means for frontal EEG delta, theta, alpha, beta, and frontal EEG asymmetry (right minus left) log power values for light- and moderate-pressure massage and vibratory stimulation groups

	Light			Moderate			Vibratory		
	Pre-	During	Post-	Pre-	During	Post-	Pre-	During	Post-
Delta (1–4Hz) trial	3.45	3.10	3.10	3.36	3.68	3.49	3.07	3.05	3.14
Theta (5–7Hz) trial	2.02	1.69	1.93	1.99	1.96	2.16	1.90	1.81	2.00
Alpha (8–12Hz) trial	3.01	2.64	2.79	3.15	2.82	2.93	3.04	2.82	3.08
Beta (13–20Hz) trial	2.32	2.13	2.41	2.41	2.20	2.28	2.36	2.27	2.39
Alpha asymmetry trial	−0.09	−0.04	−0.01	−0.32	0.00	0.01	−0.25	−0.25	−0.20

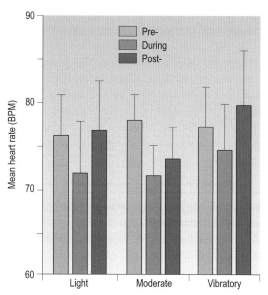

Figure 4.5 Mean heart rate in beats per minute (error bars indicate ±2 SE) for light- and moderate-pressure massage and vibratory stimulation groups.

Discussion

The moderate-pressure massage resulted in the greatest decrease in self-reported stress. The decrease in self-reported anxiety and stress is consistent with findings from several studies indicating that moderate-pressure massage therapy is effective in reducing stress and anxiety, as indicated by self-report assessments and decreases in cortisol levels.

The moderate-pressure massage therapy group exhibited both an increase in frontal EEG delta waves during the massage and a decrease in heart rate during and after the massage. Slow-wave EEG activity (delta power) is associated with lower arousal and relaxation (Niedermeyer & Lopes da Silva 1982) as are decreases in heart rate (Mok & Wong 2003). Contrary to the moderate-pressure massage, the light-pressure massage resulted in a decrease in frontal delta power during and after the massage and an increase in heart rate following the massage, suggesting increased arousal and decreased relaxation. Unlike the massage groups, the vibratory stimulation group did not exhibit any changes in slow-wave EEG activity (delta or theta), and only a marginal increase in heart rate following the stimulation.

Taken together, these findings indicate that whereas moderate-pressure massage resulted in enhanced relaxation, the light-pressure massage resulted in physiological arousal and decreased relaxation. Further, the vibratory stimulation appeared to have negligible effects on physiological levels of arousal and/or relaxation. Greater left frontal EEG alpha asymmetry is manifested during the expression of positive, approach emotions (Davidson 1998,

2000). The greatest shift towards left frontal EEG asymmetry for the moderate-pressure massage group suggests that this modality was more pleasant and relaxing than either the light-pressure massage or the vibratory stimulation.

STUDY 6: AROMATHERAPY POSITIVELY AFFECTS MOOD, EEG PATTERNS OF ALERTNESS AND MATH COMPUTATIONS

Aromas have direct effects on mood changes. These effects may be explained by the close association between the olfactory and limbic systems (see Lindsley & Holmes 1984 for reviews). Lorig & Schwartz (1987a) found, for example, that certain essential oils (lavender, spiced apple and eucalyptus) modified EEG activity including increasing relaxation as suggested by increases in alpha power. In another study Lorig and colleagues (Lorig et al 1990) found that frontal beta EEG activity increased during lavender presentation and decreased during spiced apple presentation. Parasuraman et al (1992) found that subjects exposed to a peppermint aroma were better able to sustain their attentiveness. Aromatherapy research has also shown behavioral changes including improved mood (Roberts & Williams 1992), positive affect (Miltner et al 1994), and enhanced attention and performance on visual vigilance tasks (Warm et al 1991), and decreased stress (Lorig & Schwartz 1987b).

The present study examined aromatherapy effects on feelings of relaxation, anxiety, mood and alertness and on EEG activity and math computations (Diego et al 1998). Two aromas were examined, an alerting odor (rosemary) and a relaxing odor (lavender). After the aromatherapy session the subjects who experienced the lavender aroma were expected to report less anxiety, better mood, and to show an increase in EEG power in the alpha and beta bands, suggesting increased relaxation. In contrast, subjects who were presented the rosemary aroma were expected to show greater alertness as suggested by decreased alpha and beta power and better performance on the math computations. In addition, cortisol levels were expected to decrease for both groups as they have in other relaxation studies. For example, in a previous EEG study subjects who were given massage therapy showed a decrease in frontal alpha and beta power (suggesting alertness), an increase in frontal delta power (suggesting relaxation), reported feeling better, and performed better on a cognitive task (Field et al 1996a).

Method

Participants

The subjects were 40 faculty and staff members of the University of Miami Medical School. The participants were randomly assigned to the lavender or rosemary aroma conditions. The groups did not differ on demographic variables.

Aromatherapy procedure

The aromatherapy was given by a research assistant to subjects seated in a special massage chair. Three drops of lavender or rosemary essential oil diluted to 10% concentration in grapeseed oil (provided by Aromatherapy Associates, Inc., TX, USA) were placed on a cotton dental swab and presented in a 100 ml plastic vial. The subjects held this about 3 inches from their noses for a period of 3 minutes. The participants were asked to breathe normally through their noses and sit quietly with their eyes closed.

Assessment

The assessments were conducted in the following order:

- The EEG cap was positioned on the participant's head.
- A saliva sample was taken for cortisol assay.
- The participants completed the session baseline measures, including the demographic questionnaire, the State Anxiety Inventory (STAI; Spielberger et al 1970), the Profile of Mood States (POMS; McNair et al 1971), the tense/relaxed and drowsy/alert visual analog mood scales, and the math computations.
- The aromatherapy was given.
- Immediately after the aromatherapy, the subjects completed another math computation, the POMS depression scale, the STAI to assess anxiety.
- About 20 minutes after the end of the aromatherapy session the participants provided another saliva sample for cortisol assay.

Self-report measures

The following measures were taken before and after the therapy sessions:

- POMS (McNair et al 1971).
- STAI (Spielberger et al 1970).
- Two visual analog scales (tense/relaxed and drowsy/alert) requiring the participants to circle the number (on a 10-point ordinal scale), corresponding to the way they felt at that moment. On the tense/relaxed scale a score of 0 = 'very tense' and a score of 10 = 'very relaxed.' On the drowsy/alert scale a score of 0 = 'very drowsy' and a score of 10 = 'very alert.'

Saliva samples

Saliva samples were collected and assayed for cortisol as a measure of stress that might be expected to affect alertness and performance on math computations. The samples were collected at the beginning of the therapy sessions and 20 minutes after the end of the aromatherapy session (due to the lag in cortisol change). The samples were obtained by placing a cotton dental swab dipped in sugar-free lemonade crystals along the participants' gumlines. The swab was placed in a syringe and the saliva was squeezed into a micro-centrifuge tube. The samples were assayed at Duke University Medical School.

Math computations

Before and after the aromatherapy session, participants were given math computations involving averaging a series of seven single-digit numbers. The time needed to complete the computation and the accuracy of the computation was recorded. This measure was used to determine whether the alerting effects attributed to rosemary would translate into superior performance.

EEG procedure

EEG was considered the primary dependent variable in this study as the physiological measure of relaxation and alertness. EEG was recorded for 3-minute periods prior to, during, and after the therapy sessions, with the participants' eyes closed. The EEG was recorded using a lycra stretchable cap (Electro-Cap, Inc.) that was positioned on the participant's head (Fig. 4.6).

Results

Self-report data

The analyses revealed the following (Table 4.6):

- State Anxiety scores decreased for both groups.
- Only the lavender group had significantly better mood (lower POMS scores) after the aroma session (Fig. 4.7).
- Both groups were feeling more relaxed after the aroma session.
- The rosemary group reported feeling more alert after the aroma session.
- Both groups completed the math computations faster; however, only the lavender group's accuracy scores improved.

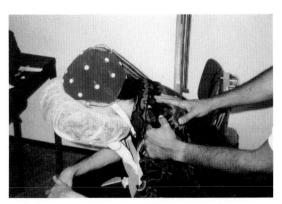

Figure 4.6   Subject in massage chair wearing EEG cap.

Table 4.6   Means for lavender and rosemary group measures

Measure	Lavender (N = 20)		Rosemary (N = 20)	
	Pre-	Post-	Pre-	Post-
State anxiety	34.32[a]	31.21	33.30[a]	26.30
Depressed mood	2.66[a]	1.16	1.45	1.74
Tense–relaxed	6.10[a]	7.68	7.00[a]	8.70
Drowsy–alert	6.16	5.95	6.00[a]	7.30
Computation time	5.14[a]	4.49	5.23[a]	4.52
Computation accuracy	2.55[a]	3.10	2.25	2.50

[a]Significant differences between adjacent numbers.

Table 4.7   Frontal log power values

	Pre-	During	Post-
		Alpha (8–12Hz)	
Lavender	3.07[a]	3.40[a]	3.72[b]
Rosemary	4.16[a]	3.74[b]	3.72[b]
		Beta 1 (13–20Hz)	
Lavender	0.57[a]	0.79[a]	0.96[a]
Rosemary	1.07[a]	0.96[b]	1.14[a]
		Beta 2 (21–30Hz)	
Lavender	−0.17[a]	0.06[a]	0.27[b]
Rosemary	0.53	0.47[a]	0.80[b]

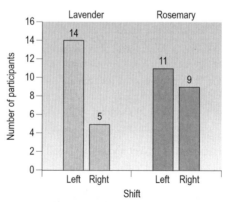

Figure 4.7   Number of participants who shifted to left frontal EEG (less depressed) or right frontal EEG (more depressed) when smelling lavender or rosemary aromas.

- Frontal alpha power increased after lavender presentation, suggesting increased drowsiness, while frontal alpha power decreased during and after the rosemary, suggesting increased alertness (Table 4.7).
- Frontal beta power increased after lavender and rosemary presentation, suggesting drowsiness.

Discussion

The fact that the lavender group reported feeling more relaxed, and the increase in beta power supports previous findings on lavender's ability to increase frontal beta power (Lorig et al 1990), promote drowsiness (Buchbauer et al 1991) and induce sleep (van Toller 1988). The rosemary findings support the belief that rosemary is an alerting aroma (van Toller 1988). The increase in frontal beta 2 power immediately after rosemary aroma was removed suggests that its alerting effect might be short-lived.

The math computation results suggest that although both groups performed the computations faster after the aroma session, only the lavender group showed improved accuracy on math computations following the sessions. This finding was surprising because the lavender group did not show the enhanced alertness EEG pattern that the rosemary group showed. Perhaps as reflected in both self-report and EEG data the lavender group was more relaxed and thus better able to concentrate. This and previous research indicate that aromas can effect psychological and physiological changes. Further research is needed on the underlying mechanisms of these effects.

References

Buchbauer B, Jirovetz L, Jager W, et al 1991 Aromatherapy: evidence for sedative effects of the essential oils of lavender after inhalation. Naturforsch 46:1067–1072.

Cigales M, Field T, Lundy B, et al 1997 Massage enhances recovery from habituation in normal infants. Infant Behavior and Development 20:29–34.

Conners CK 1997 Conners Rating Scales—Revised; technical manual. Multi-Health Systems, North Tonawanda, NY.

Davidson RJ 1998 Anterior electrophysiological asymmetries, emotion, and depression: conceptual and methodological conundrums. Psychophysiology 35:607–614.

Davidson RJ 2000 Affective style, psychopathology, and resilience: brain mechanisms and plasticity. American Psychologist 55:1196–1214.

Dawson G, Galpert L 1990 Mothers' use of imitative play for facilitating social responsiveness and toy play in young autistic children. Development and Psychopathology 2:151–162.

Diego M, Jones N, Field T, et al 1998 Aromatherapy positively affects mood, EEG patterns of alertness and math computations. International Journal of Neuroscience 96:217–224.

Diego M, Field T, Sanders C, et al 2004 Massage therapy of moderate and light pressure and vibrator effects on EEG and heart rate. International Journal of Neuroscience 114:31–44.

Eaton WO, McKeen NA, Lam CS 1988 Instrumented motor activity measurement of the young infant in the home: factor structure, reliability, and criterion validity. Infant Behavior and Development 11:375–378.

Escalona A, Field T, Singer-Strunck R, et al 2001 Brief Report: Improvements in the behavior of children with autism following massage therapy. Journal of Autism and Developmental Disorders 31:513–516.

Field T 1990 Newborn behavior, vagal tone and catecholamine activity in cocaine exposed infants. Symposium presented at the International Society of Infant Studies, April. Montreal, Canada.

Field T 1995 Touch in early development. Erlbaum, New Jersey.

Field T 1998 Massage therapy effects. American Psychologist 53:1270–1281.

Field T, Morrow C, Valdeon C, et al 1992 Massage reduces anxiety in child and adolescent psychiatric patients. Journal of the American Academy of Child Adolescent Psychiatry 30:125–131.

Field T, Harding J, Soliday B, et al 1994 Touching in infant, toddler, and preschool nurseries. Early Child Development and Care 98:113–120.

Field T, Ironson G, Pickens J, et al 1996a Massage therapy reduces anxiety and enhances EEG pattern of alertness and math computations. International Journal of Neuroscience 86:197–205.

Field T, Kilmer T, Hernandez-Reif M, et al 1996b Preschool children's sleep and wake behavior: effects of massage therapy. Early Child Development & Care 120:39–44.

Field T, Hernandez-Reif M, Seligman S, et al 1997a Juvenile rheumatoid arthritis benefits from massage therapy. Journal of Pediatric Psychology 22:607–617.

Field T, Lasko D, Mundy P, et al 1997b Autistic children's attentiveness and responsivity improve after touch therapy. Journal of Autism and Developmental Disorders 27:333–338.

Field T, Quintino O, Henteleff T, et al 1997a Job stress reduction therapies. Alternative Therapies 3:54–56.

Field TM, Quintino O, Hernandez-Reif M, et al 1998 Adolescents with attention deficit hyperactivity disorder benefit from massage therapy. Adolescence 33:103–108.

Hart S, Field T, Hernandez-Reif M, et al 1998 Preschoolers' cognitive performance improves following massage. Early Childhood Development and Care 143:59–64.

Hernandez-Reif M, Field T, Thimas E 1999 ADHD benefits from Tai Chi. Journal of Bodywork and Movement Therapies 5:120–123.

Hovind H, Nielsen SL 1974 Effect of massage on blood flow in skeletal muscle. Scandinavian Journal of Rehabilitation Medicine 6(2):74–77.

Khilnani S, Field T, Hernandez-Reif M, et al 2003 Massage therapy improves mood and behavior of students with attention-deficit/hyperactivity disorder. Adolescence 152:623–638.

Klinger LG, Dawson G 1996 Autistic disorder. In: Mash EJ, Barkley RA (eds) Child psychopathology. Guilford Press, New York, pp. 311–339.

Lecuyer R 1989 Habituation and attention, novelty and cognition: where is the continuity? Human Development 32:148–157.

Lindsley DF, Holmes JE 1984 Basic human neuropsychology. Elsevier, New York.

Lorig TS, Schwartz GE 1987a EEG activity during fine fragrance administration. Psychophysiology 24:599.

Lorig TS, Schwartz GE 1987b EEG activity during relaxation and fool imagery. Psychophysiology 24:599.

Lorig TA, Schwartz GE 1988 Brain and odor: I. Alteration of human EEG by odor administration. Psychobiology 16:281–284.

Lorig TS, Herman KB, Schwartz GE, et al 1990 EEG activity during administration of low-concentration odors. Bulletin of the Psychonomic Society 28:405–408.

Lundeberg T, Nordemar R, Ottoson D 1984 Pain alleviation by vibratory stimulation. Pain 20:25–44.

McKechnie AA, Wilson F, Watson N, et al 1983 Anxiety states: a preliminary report on the value of connective tissue massage. Journal of Psychosomatic Research 27:125–129.

McNair DM, Lorr M, Droppleman LF 1971 Profile of Mood States. Educational and Industrial Testing Service, San Diego.

Mesibov GB, Adams LW, Klinger LG 1997 Autism: understanding the disorder. Plenum Press, New York.

Miltner W, Matjak M, Diekmann H, et al 1994 Emotional qualities of odors and their influence on the startle reflex in humans. Psychophysiology 31:107–110.

Mok E, Wong KY 2003 Effects of music on patient anxiety. AORN Journal 77:396–397.

Niedermeyer E, Lopes da Silva F 1982 Electroencephalography. Basic principles, clinical applications and related fields. Urban and Schwarzenberg, Baltimore.

Nunez PL 2000 Toward a quantitative description of large-scale neocortical dynamic function and EEG. Behavioral & Brain Sciences 23:371–437.

Ottoson D, Ekblom A, Hansson P 1981 Vibratory stimulation for the relief of pain of dental origin. Pain 10:37–45.

Parasuraman R, Warm JS, Dember WN 1992 Effects of olfactory stimulation on skin conductance and event-related brain potentials during visual sustained attention. Fragrance Research Fund Ltd, New York.

Porges SW 1997 Emotion: an evolutionary by-product of the neural regulation of the autonomic nervous system. In: Carter CS, Kirkpatrick B, Lederhendler II (eds) The integrative neurobiology of affiliation. New York Academy of Sciences, New York, pp. 62–77.

Porges SW 1998 Love: an emergent property of the mammalian autonomic nervous system. Psychoneuroendocrinology 23:837–861.

Porges SW 1991 Vagal tone: a mediator of affect. In: Garber JA, Dodge KA (eds) The development of affect regulation and dysregulation. Cambridge University Press, New York, pp. 111–128.

Rieppi R, Greenhill LL, Ford RE, et al 2002 Socioeconomic status as a moderator of ADHD treatment outcomes. Journal of the American Academy of Child and Adolescent Psychiatry 41:269–277.

Roberts A, Williams JMG 1992 The effect of olfactory stimulation on fluency, vividness of imagery and associated mood: a preliminary study. British Journal of Medical Psychology 65:197–199.

Rogers S 1999 An examination of the imitation deficit in autism. In: Nadel J, Butterworth G (eds) Imitation in infancy. Cambridge studies in cognitive perceptual development. Cambridge University Press, New York, pp 290–302.

Scafidi F, Field T, Schanberg S, et al 1990 Massage stimulates growth in preterm infants: a replication. Infant Behavior and Development 13:167–188.

Schopler E, Reichler R 1979 Individualized assessment and treatment for autistic and developmentally disabled children: Vol I. Psychoeducational profile. University Park Press, Baltimore.

Shoemaker JK, Tiidus PM, Mader R 1997 Failure of manual massage to alter limb blood flow: measures by Doppler ultrasound. Medicine and Science in Sports and Exercise 29(5):610–614.

Shulman KR, Jones GE 1996 The effectiveness of massage therapy intervention on reducing anxiety in the workplace. Journal of Applied Behavioral Science 32:160–173.

Spencer T, Biederman J, Coffey B, et al 2002 A double-blind comparison of desipramine and placebo in children and adolescents with chronic tic disorder and comorbid attention-deficit/hyperactivity disorder. Archives of General Psychiatry 59:649–656.

Spielberger C, Gorsuch R, Lushene R 1970 The State Trait Anxiety Inventory. Consulting Psychologists Press, Palo Alto, CA.

Sullivan SJ, Williams LR, Seaborne DE, et al 1991 Effects of massage on alpha motoneuron excitability Physical Therapy 71(8):555–560.

Tsai L 1992 Medical treatment in autism. In: Berkell DE (ed.). Autism identification, education, and treatment. Lawrence Erlbaum Associates Inc, New Jersey, pp. 151–184.

van Toller S 1988 Emotion and the brain. In: van Toller S, Dodd GH (eds) Perfumery: the psychology and biology of fragrance. Chapman & Hall, London, pp 56–98.

Warm JS, Dember WN, Parasuraman R 1991 Effects of olfactory stimulation on performance and stress in a visual sustained attention task. Journal of the Society of Cosmetic Chemists 42:199–210.

Wechsler D 1989 Wechsler Preschool and Primary Scale of Intelligence—Revised. Harcourt Brace Jovanovitch, San Antonio.

Chapter 5

Decreasing depression and aggression

EEG in the frontal region of the brain is typically more activated on the right side in depressed individuals. During some treatments, EEG has been noted to shift to the left side, which is more responsible for processing positive emotions like happiness. In the following group of studies, various therapies including aroma, music, and massage have been noted to shift the predominant right frontal EEG activity to symmetry (in the center) or towards the left frontal region (a positive shift in EEG). In the first study, depressed individuals who were showing right frontal EEG activity prior to the aroma session were noted to shift towards the left following the presentation of a lavender aroma (Diego et al 1998). In the second study, massage and music were provided to depressed individuals (Field et al 1998). In both of these conditions, the depressed individuals were noted to experience a shift from right to left frontal EEG activation. In the third study, massage therapy was notably effective with aggressive adolescents (Diego et al 2002). Brief chair massages decreased their aggressive behavior.

STUDY 1: EEG DURING LAVENDER AND ROSEMARY EXPOSURE IN INFANTS OF DEPRESSED AND NON-DEPRESSED MOTHERS

Depressed adults show greater relative right frontal electroencephalographic (EEG) asymmetry than non-depressed adults (Davidson 1998). A similar pattern of greater relative right frontal EEG asymmetry has been observed in infants born to depressed mothers (Field et al 1995, Jones et al 1997), and shifts towards greater relative right frontal EEG asymmetry have been observed in infants exhibiting negative affect (Fox & Davidson 1988). Human infants exposed to lavender exhibit lower saliva cortisol levels after a heel lance than controls who received no odor, suggesting that lavender has calming effects on infants (Kawakami et al 1997). In a study on adults, exposure to lavender and rosemary altered EEG patterns in a positive direction and improved mood (Diego et al 1998). If aromas like lavender and rosemary are perceived by young infants as positive stimuli, then this might be reflected in their EEG pattern, as has been shown for other sensory stimuli, and in their facial expressions, as has been shown for other pleasant odors.

The purpose of the present study was to investigate infant affective and frontal EEG responses to rosemary and lavender aromas. Based on adult findings, we expected that exposure to both lavender and rosemary aromas would cause a shift towards greater relative left frontal EEG asymmetry in newborns of both depressed and non-depressed mothers. Both groups of infants were also expected to exhibit greater positive affect in response to the aromas.

Method

Participants

Forty-five mothers were recruited from an ongoing longitudinal study on the effects of maternal depression on infants. Infants were randomly assigned to receive either a lavender or a rosemary aroma. Group inclusion was based on mothers' scores on the Center for Epidemiological Studies Depression Scale (CES-D) (Radloff 1977), with the depressed group scoring >16 on the CES-D and the non-depressed group scoring <12. Infants were on average 19 days old.

Procedure and design

Upon arrival at the EEG laboratory, mothers read and signed a consent form approved by the university's human subjects committee. The newborns were fed and changed prior to testing. Subsequently, the infants were reclined in an infant seat and EEG and electro-oculogram (EOG) electrodes were attached. The EEG and video recording began when the newborn was quiet and alert and were recorded continuously during a 2-minute baseline phase, followed by a 2-minute odor-exposure phase.

The essential oils of rosemary and lavender (donated by Aromatherapy Associates, FL, USA) were diluted in odorless grapeseed oil to form a 10% v/v solution. Three drops of the solution were poured on a sterile dental swab and placed in a pierced metal container. The odor emanated for 2 minutes from the metal container, which, at the beginning of the odor trial, was suspended manually approximately 15 cm above the infant's head and out of the infant's view. To contain the aroma, the metal container was stored in a sealed jar before and after the exposure phase.

Infants' facial expressions were videotaped. The video was later coded for negative affect, head turns, lip-licking, and nose wrinkling, as these measures have been coded by researchers who study infant smell perception (Mennella & Beauchamp 1993). Behaviors were coded as they occurred during sequential 10-second blocks. The total number of time sample units that a behavior occurred was divided by the total number of time sample units to yield percentage time that behavior occurred. The percentage time for baseline was subtracted from the 'during odor' percentage to yield difference scores for each behavior. Prior to videotape recording, 9-mm gold-cup electrodes were placed on the infants' scalp at two mid-frontal sites. Asymmetry scores were computed using natural log scores. The asymmetry score is a difference score reflecting power in one hemisphere relative to power in the homologous site in the contralateral hemisphere, with negative scores reflecting greater relative right frontal EEG asymmetry and positive scores reflecting greater relative left frontal EEG asymmetry.

Results

The two odors did not have different effects. Thus, we compared the EEG asymmetry scores and the behavioral data across aromas for the depressed and non-depressed groups. Data analyses revealed that newborns of depressed mothers were more likely to show a shift towards greater relative left frontal EEG asymmetry from baseline to the exposure phase than newborns of non-depressed mothers (see Fig. 5.1). Data analyses revealed that head turning increased in the depressed group versus the non-depressed group. Correlation analyses revealed that the shift in frontal EEG asymmetry changes was related to head turning, and head turning in turn was related to lip-licking.

Discussion

The shift toward greater relative left frontal EEG asymmetry by newborns of depressed mothers when exposed to rosemary and lavender aromas is a pattern associated with positive affect and response to positive stimuli. Why these odors only elicited differential EEG patterns for newborns of depressed mothers is not known. Perhaps newborns of depressed mothers have higher sensory thresholds. If the odors were strong and the infants of depressed mothers had a higher olfactory threshold than those of non-depressed mothers,

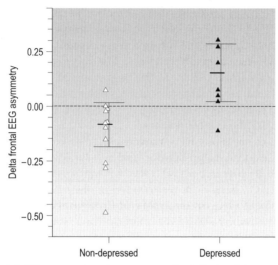

Figure 5.1 Frontal EEG asymmetry change scores for infants of depressed and non-depressed mothers.

then the odors might not have been aversive to the depressed group but aversive to the non-depressed group.

Studies on depressed adults suggest that they have odor identification deficits, possibly because of their higher thresholds. Thus, strong odors may be perceived as pleasant by newborns of depressed mothers, who have higher olfactory thresholds than newborns of non-depressed mothers. To test this hypothesis, a future study might examine the effects of rosemary and lavender at different concentrations on the EEG of infants of depressed and non-depressed mothers.

Newborns of depressed mothers showed greater head turning during the odor exposure. Olko & Turkewitz (2001) noted that pleasant odors (as determined by adults), but not unpleasant odors, elicited head turns toward the scent. These findings suggest a relationship between head turning and left frontal EEG asymmetry and are consistent with the significant relationship found between head turning and frontal EEG asymmetry in the infant study. Future studies should examine the direction of head turning to test this hypothesis, perhaps by presenting the odor to the infant's right or left side to see if the infant turns toward or away from the odor.

STUDY 2: MASSAGE AND MUSIC THERAPIES ATTENUATE FRONTAL EEG ASYMMETRY IN DEPRESSED ADOLESCENTS

EEG asymmetry, specifically greater relative right frontal activation, is associated with negative affect. Depressed adults show stable patterns of this asymmetry. The present study assessed the effects of massage therapy and music therapy on frontal EEG asymmetry in depressed adolescents (Jones & Field 1999).

Massage therapy has led to a reduction in anxiety, depression, and stress hormone in depressed adolescent mothers (Field et al 1996a). Further, music has been found to shift frontal EEG patterns toward symmetry in adolescents who were depressed (Field et al 1998), and massage therapy has attenuated EEG asymmetry in infants of depressed mothers (Jones et al 1998). The latter findings are surprising given that frontal EEG asymmetry is believed to be stable (Tomarken et al 1992). For example, previously depressed adults were found to have greater relative right frontal EEG activation even though they no longer showed behavioral symptoms (Henriques & Davidson 1990), suggesting that it is a physiological marker for depression, independent of depressed behavior. The present study investigated the effects of massage therapy in a sample of depressed adolescents with greater relative right frontal EEG activation.

Method

Participants

Thirty adolescents were randomly assigned to massage and music groups. Adolescents' scores on the CES-D (Center for Epidemiologic Studies Depression Scale; Radloff, 1977) were >16, indicating depression. The adolescents also met DISC (Diagnostic Interview Schedule for Children; Robins et al 1981) criteria for dysthymia or major depressive disorder. In addition, their baseline EEG patterns indicated greater relative right frontal activation.

Procedure

EEG   3-minute EEG recordings were obtained prior to, during, and after the massage/music sessions. A stretchable lycra EEG cap was placed on the participant's head. EEG asymmetry scores were computed. Negative scores indicate greater relative right hemisphere activation, whereas positive scores indicate greater relative left hemisphere activation (Davidson 1988).

Massage   Massage therapy was provided by a professional massage therapist for 15 minutes. The fully-clothed adolescents sat in a special massage chair while receiving a massage consisting of long, broad strokes, using moderate pressure, administered to the back, arms, hands, and neck (Field et al 1996b).

Music   Music therapy involved listening to 15 minutes of uplifting rock music. This music had previously been selected by a group of adolescents who were similar to the study sample (Field et al 1998). The songs included 'Straight Up' by Paula Abdul (upbeat dance song), 'Nasty' by Janet Jackson (upbeat dance song), 'Vision of Love' by Mariah Carey (slow love ballad), 'Greatest Love of All' by Whitney Houston (slow inspirational ballad), and

'Keep the Faith' by Michael Jackson (moderate tempo, inspirational). The adolescents wore headphones to listen to this high-fidelity music.

Results

T-tests revealed that both the massage and the music therapies produced significant attenuation of frontal EEG asymmetry: from pre-session to during session, and from pre-session to post-session (see Fig. 5.2).

Discussion

In the present study efforts to reduce frontal EEG asymmetry were successful. Greater relative right frontal EEG activation was significantly lessened using both massage therapy and music therapy (Fig. 5.3). The results suggest that various relaxation techniques can be used to alter EEG patterns (Field 1995). Future studies should investigate whether these therapies can decrease the vulnerability to psychological disorders.

STUDY 3: AGGRESSIVE ADOLESCENTS BENEFIT FROM MASSAGE THERAPY

Aggressive behavior among adolescents has become a major public health problem (Centers for Disease Control and Prevention 2001). Aggression, which can be defined as 'destructive behavior with intent to inflict harm or

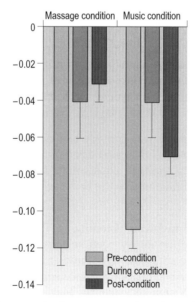

Figure 5.2   Frontal EEG asymmetry for massage and music conditions.

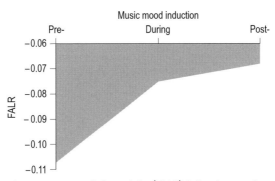

Figure 5.3 Frontal asymmetry on left or right (FALR) following music mood induction.

physical damage' (Marwick 1996, p. 90), remains one of the most difficult problems to study and treat in adolescents (Malone et al 1994). Due to lack of effectiveness of any single behavioral or cognitive treatment for all types of aggression (stemming from the complex mechanisms underlying aggressive behavior), and the unpleasant side-effects of psychotropic drugs, complementary therapies are being investigated, such as training in aikido (a martial art similar to karate or judo), as a means of reducing aggressiveness in youth (Delva 1995). Although massage therapy reduces depression and anxiety, factors noted to be related to aggression, the effects of massage therapy on aggression have not been studied previously. The present study evaluated the effects of 5 weeks of massage therapy versus relaxation therapy on aggressive adolescents (Diego et al 2002).

Method

Participants

The participants were recruited from a child and adolescent psychiatry outpatient clinic at a major urban university hospital if they met the following criteria:

- score of 10 or higher on the behavior component of the Overt Aggression Scale (OAS)
- no acute suicidal threat
- no psychosis
- no mental retardation
- medically stable
- able to understand and communicate.

The participants were then stratified by age and aggression subtype and randomly assigned to a massage therapy or a progressive muscle relaxation/attention control group, before their first visit.

Procedure

Massage therapy   The participants in the massage therapy group received two 20-minute chair massage therapy sessions per week for 5 weeks. The professional massage therapist (a different therapist each session) administered a standard massage procedure with the adolescent sitting fully clothed in the special massage chair. This consisted of long, broad stroking with moderate pressure to the back: (1) compression to the back parallel to the spine from the shoulders to the base of the spine, (2) compression to the entire back adding rocking, (3) trapezius squeeze, (4) finger pressure on the shoulder, (5) finger pressure along the length of the spine and back, and (6) circular stroking of the hips; arms: (1) arms dropped to the side with arms kneaded from shoulder to lower arm, and (2) pressing down on upper and lower arms; hands: (1) entire hands massaged and pulling of fingers, (2) the fleshy part of the palm pressed between the thumb and index finger for 15–20 seconds, and (3) pulling of the arms in both lateral and superior directions; neck: (1) kneading area of cervical vertebrae, (2) finger pressure along base of skull and along side of neck, (3) scalp massage, and (4) pressing down on trapezius with finger pressure and squeezing continuing down the arms.

Relaxation therapy   The participants in this group were guided through two 20-minute progressive muscle relaxation sessions per week for 5 weeks by a researcher or a massage therapist (a different therapist each session). The progressive muscle relaxation routine developed by Jacobsen (1929) consisted of a calm and soothing voice instructing the adolescents, who were sitting in the massage chair, to successively tense and relax each of the major muscle groups in the same progression as the massage procedure as follows: back, arms, hands, and neck.

Assessments

On the first and last days of the study, prior to the therapy, the parents/legal guardians were asked to complete a demographic questionnaire, the OAS, and the Child Behavior Checklist. The adolescents were asked to complete the SCL-90R, and the State Anxiety Inventory for Children (STAI-C).

Overt Aggression Scale (OAS)   Parents were asked to complete the OAS, a 20-item checklist on aggressive behavior (Yudofsky et al 1986), verbal aggression (i.e. curses viciously, uses foul language in anger, makes moderate threats to self or others), aggression against objects (i.e. breaks objects, smashes windows), aggression against self (i.e. small cuts or bruises, minor burns), and aggression against others (i.e. attacks others, causing mild–moderate physical injury).

Child Behavior Checklist (CBCL)   The CBCL (Achenbach 1994, Achenbach & Edelbrock 1987) is a 100-item questionnaire. The parents only completed the 47 questions on the aggressive (i.e. physically attacks people), delinquent (i.e. disobedient at home), and hostility (i.e. impulsive or acts without think-ing) subscales.

SCL-90R   The SCL-90R (Derogatis 1983) is a 90-item questionnaire. For the purposes of this study, the adolescents completed only the items on the hostil-ity subscale. The SCL-90R consists of simple statements such as 'Having urges to break or smash things', followed by five choices of severity (0 = not at all to 4 = extremely).

State Anxiety Inventory for Children (STAI-C)   The STAI-C (Spielberger 1973) is designed to assess the transitory level of anxiety in children and young adolescents. It consists of 20 items each with a choice of three levels of severity (i.e. 'I feel very nervous', '. . . nervous', '. . . not nervous').

Results

Data analyses revealed the following (Tables 5.1 and 5.2):

- only the massage therapy group showed a significant decrease in OAS aggression (Fig. 5.4)
- only the massage therapy group showed a significant decrease in CBCL aggression scores
- only the massage therapy group showed a significant decrease in hostility scores on the SCL-90R
- only the massage therapy group showed a significant decrease in state anxiety on the STAI-C and only after the first session.

Table 5.1   Means for long-term massage versus relaxation therapy effects

	Massage		Relaxation	
Type of aggression	Day 1	Day 10	Day 1	Day 10
OAS Total	27.67[a]	22.11[b]	23.75[a]	22.25[a]
CBCL (aggression)	15.22[a]	13.11[b]	16.50[a]	15.63[a]
CBCL (delinquent)	9.78[a]	8.89[a]	9.13[a]	7.88[a]
SCL-90R (hostility)	12.67[a]	10.78[b]	9.50[a]	7.75[a]

[a,b]Significant Day1/Day10 differences between means.

Table 5.2   Means for immediate effects of massage versus relaxation therapy

	Massage		Relaxation	
	Pre-	Post-	Pre-	Post-
STAI-C Day 1	37.22[a]	31.89[b]	35.25[a]	34.13[a]
STAI-C Day 10	35.89[a]	27.22[b]	33.75[a]	31.50[a]

[a,b]Significant pre-/post- differences between means.

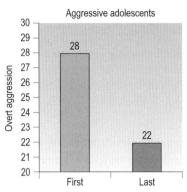

Figure 5.4 Overt aggression scores on first day and last day of massage therapy study.

Discussion

The adolescents who received massage therapy reported feeling less anxious after the first 20-minute session of treatment, but participants receiving progressive muscle relaxation did not. This is consistent with previous studies showing that, for children and adolescents, anxiety and stress hormone levels decrease following massage therapy (Field et al 1992). The reduction in aggression and hostility noted by the adolescents who received massage therapy, as well as their parents, may relate to the reduction noted in their anxiety levels and a reduction in stress hormone levels noted in previous massage therapy studies (Field et al 1992, 1996b). They may have had lower arousal levels and therefore better control over their impulsive and reactive behavior. Further studies should document the effects of massage therapy on aggressive adolescents' relationships and their neurochemical and psychophysiological responses to this therapy.

References

Achenbach T 1994 Child Behavior Checklist and related instruments. In: Maruish ME, et al (eds) The use of psychologial testing for treatment planning and outcome assessment. Lawrence Erlbaum Associates, Mahwah, NJ, pp. 517–549.

Achenbach T, Edelbrock C 1987 Manual for the youth self-report and profile. University of Vermont Department of Psychiatry, Burlington, VT.

Centers for Disease Control and Prevention 2001 Deaths: final data for 1999. National Vital Statistics Report 49(8).

Davidson R 1988 EEG measures of cerebral activation: conceptual and methodological issues. International Journal of Neuroscience 39:71–89.

Davidson R 1998 Anterior electrophysiological asymmetries, emotion, and depression: conceptual and methodological conundrums. Psychophysiology 35:607–614.

Delva T 1995 Does brief aikido training reduce aggression of youth? Perceptual and Motor Skill 80:297–298.

Derogatis LR 1983 SCL-90R, administration, scoring and procedures manual, 2nd edn. Clinical Psychometric Research, Townson, MD.

Diego M, Jones N, Field T, et al 1998 Aromatherapy positively affects mood, EEG patterns of alertness and math computations. International Journal of Neuroscience 96:217–224.

Diego M, Field T, Hernandez-Reif M, et al 2002 Aggressive adolescents benefit from massage therapy. Adolescence 37:597–607.

Field T 1995 Infants of depressed mothers. Infant Behavior and Development 18:1–13.

Field T, Morrow C, Valdeon C, et al 1992 Massage reduces anxiety in child and adolescent psychiatric patients. Journal of the American Academy of Child and Adolescent Psychiatry 31(1):125–131.

Field T, Fox N, Pickens J, et al 1995 Relative right frontal EEG activation in 3- to 6-month-old infants of depressed mothers. Special Section: Parental depression and distress: implications for development in infancy, childhood, and adolescence. Developmental Psychology 31:358–363.

Field T, Grizzle N, Scafidi F, et al 1996a Massage and relaxation therapies' effects on depressed adolescent mothers. Adolescence 31:903–911.

Field T, Ironson G, Scafidi F, et al 1996b Massage therapy reduces anxiety and enhances EEG patterns of alertness and math computations. International Journal of Neuroscience 56:197–205.

Field T, Martinez A, Nawrocki T, et al 1998 Music shifts frontal EEG in depressed adolescents. Adolescence 33:109–116.

Fox N, Davidson R 1988 Patterns of brain electrical activity during the expression of discrete emotions in ten month old infants. Developmental Psychology 24:230–236.

Henriques J, Davidson R 1990 Regional brain electrical asymmetries discriminate between previously depressed and healthy control subjects. Journal of Abnormal Psychology 99:22–31.

Jacobsen 1929 Progressive relaxation. University of Chicago Press, Chicago.

Jones NA, Field T 1999 Massage and music therapies attenuate frontal EEG asymmetry in depressed adolescents. Adolescence 34:529–534.

Jones NA, Field T, Fox NA, et al 1997 Right frontal EEG patterns in 1-month-old infants of depressed mothers. Development and Psychopathology 9:491–505.

Jones N, Field T, Davalos M 1998 Massage therapy attenuates right frontal EEG asymmetry in one-month-old infants of depressed mothers. Infant Behavior and Development 21:527–530.

Kawakami K, Takai-Kawakami K, Okazaki Y, et al 1997 The effect of odors on human infants under stress. Infant Behavior and Development 20(4):531–535.

Malone R, Luebbert J, Pena-Ariet M, et al 1994 The Overt Aggression Scale in a study of lithium in aggressive conduct disorder. Psychopharmacology Bulletin 30(2):215–218.

Marwick C 1996 Childhood aggression needs definition, therapy. Journal of the American Medical Association 275(2):90.

Mennella J, Beauchamp G 1993 Early flavor experiences: when do they start? Zero to Three 14:1–7.

Olko C, Turkewitz G 2001 Cerebral asymmetry of emotion and its relationship to olfactory in infancy. Laterality 6(1):29–37.

Radloff L 1977 The CES-D Scale: a self-report symptoms scale to detect depression in a community sample. American Journal of Psychiatry 137:1081–1083.

Robins L, Helzer J, Croughan J, et al 1981 National Institute of Mental Health Diagnostic Interview Schedule. Archives of General Psychiatry 38:381–390.

Spielberger CD 1973 Manual for the State-Trait Anxiety Inventory for Children. Consulting Psychologists Press, Palo Alto.

Tomarken A, Davidson R, Wheeler R, et al 1992 Psychometric properties of resting anterior EEG asymmetry: temporal stability and internal consistency. Psychophysiology 29:576–592.

Yudofsky SC, Silver JM, Jackson W, et al 1986 The Overt Aggression Scale for the objective rating of verbal and physical aggression. American Journal of Psychiatry 143(1):35–39.

Chapter 6

Improving neuromuscular function

Massage therapy might be expected to improve range of motion and increase muscle strength inasmuch as it involves direct application of pressure on the muscle tissue. In at least five studies, we have demonstrated an increase in range of motion and/or increased strength and improved neuromuscular function. In the first study on dancers, we were able to show that massage therapy increased shoulder abduction (Leivadi et al 1999). In another study on spinal cord patients, we were able to show enhanced muscle strength in the upper limbs in those who were experiencing paralysis in the lower half of their body (paraplegia) (Diego et al 2002). In a study on cerebral palsy, massage therapy led to a decrease in hypertonicity in the arms and legs (Hernandez-Reif et al 2005a), and, in Down's syndrome, a decrease in hypotonicity in the arms and legs (Hernandez-Reif et al 2005b). In a study on

Parkinson's disease, which is generally accompanied by uncontrolled, disorganized facial movements, we were able to show that exerting pressure against the skin in the form of massage therapy led to a reduction in these uncontrolled movements (Hernandez-Reif et al 2002).

STUDY 1: MASSAGE THERAPY AND RELAXATION EFFECTS ON UNIVERSITY DANCE STUDENTS

Movement in dance is often performed at the extremes of range of motion and thus can be stressful for the body as muscles are shortened or stretched to lengths that provide for suboptimal contraction and power. Traditionally, improved range of motion is achieved through physical therapy, strength training, and resistance and stretching exercises. Various forms of massage therapy have been considered for improving range of motion (O'Rourke 1998, Stikeleather 1991, Twomey 1992).

This study examined massage therapy for decreasing stress hormones and potential stressors such as anxiety, and neck, shoulder and back pain related to dancing. Massage therapy was also expected to improve mood and range of motion (Leivadi et al 1999).

Method

Thirty female adult dance majors were recruited from a university dance conservatory. The participants were randomly assigned to a massage (N = 15) or relaxation therapy (N = 15) group.

Massage therapy   Those assigned to massage therapy received 30-minute sessions twice a week for 5 consecutive weeks. The sessions were conducted by different trained massage therapists to ensure that their skills were evenly distributed across the pool of participants. Massages were performed at the physical therapy facility of the Dance Conservatory during the mid-afternoon and focused on the upper torso. The therapy consisted of moderate-to-firm pressure, long smooth stroking motions, rocking, pressing, and stretching. With the dancer in a prone position, the massage progressed in the following sequence: (1) firm strokes gliding along and slightly stretching the skin of the neck, back and shoulders to warm tissues, (2) short up-and-down and side-to-side strokes (friction) sequentially down either side of the spinal column to focus on muscles and tendons beneath the skin from the head to the tailbone, then continuing to the sides, along the upper edge of the hip bones, (3) squeezing and lifting the skin and muscle along either side of the vertebral column, around the sides of the body, along the shoulder tops and the back part of the armpit, and below the arms, (4) up-and-down and side-to-side strokes in sequence along the upper and outer edges of the collar bones and the wing bones, (5) stretch of the scapular muscles by lifting the scapula away from the rib cage, (6) slow and firm pressure on the muscles away from the vertebral column, moving sequentially from head to sacrum on one side and then the other, (7) gliding of fingers or thumbs slowly and very firmly down the neck and along the top of the shoulder, following the fibers of the upper trapezius muscles, continuing down the neck and across the upper back and progressing to the bottom of the scapula, repeating on the other side.

Finally, the massage concluded with the participant lying on her side and progressed in the following sequence for each side: (1) firm pressure on the muscles along the rib cage and chest waiting for a release of tension before moving on, (2) lifting, squeezing, stretching and 'unrolling' the bulk of the chest muscles avoiding breast tissue, continuing with friction sequentially along the available edges of the sternum and clavicle, (3) slowly circling the arm up by the head, behind the back, and down along the side while gently pressing into the chest and side muscles to relax and stretch them, (4) pressing into the lateral neck muscles attaching along the side of the neck; squeezing and releasing tension in the sternocleidomastoid (SCM) muscle, and (5) reversing the circling of the arm and using the weight of the arm to stretch middle back and chest muscles.

Relaxation therapy   A relaxation group, as opposed to a standard control group, was used for comparison. This group controlled for potential placebo effects, or potential improvement related to the increased attention given to the massage participants. The participants listened via earphones to instructions on how to conduct progressive muscle relaxation sessions while lying quietly on a mat. A session lasted 30 minutes and consisted of tensing and relaxing large muscle groups starting with the feet and progressing to the calves, thighs, hands, arms, back and face. The dancers were asked to conduct these sessions twice a week for 5 weeks.

Assessments of immediate effects

State Anxiety Inventory (STAI) (Spielberger et al 1970)   The STAI was administered to assess anxiety levels. The questionnaire consists of 20 items and assesses how the subject feels at that moment in terms of severity.

Profile of Mood States (POMS) (McNair et al 1971)   The POMS is a five-point adjective-rating scale asking subjects to describe how well an adjective describes his/her feelings for the previous week. The questionnaire, which includes items such as helpless or gloomy, consists of 20 items measuring depression and anxiety.

VITAS (VITAS Healthcare Corporation, FL, USA)   Participants completed pre-/post-session pain scales, with reference to neck and back pain, on the first and last day of the study. Pain perception was rated on a Visual Analog Scale (VAS) ranging from 0 (no pain) to 10 (worst possible pain) and anchored with five faces. The faces, located at two-point intervals, range from very happy (0), to happy (2), contented (4), somewhat distressed (6), distressed (8) and very distressed (10). Highly acceptable scores for criterion-related validity were established by correlating the VITAS with sleep disturbance, since body pain has been associated with difficulty sleeping (Hertz et al 1992, Smith et al 1990).

Salivary cortisol   Saliva samples were collected and assayed for cortisol levels as a measure of stress. The samples were obtained at the beginning of the massage therapy or relaxation session and 20 minutes after the session on the first and last days of the study. Due to a 20-minute lagtime in cortisol changes, saliva samples always reflect responses to stimulation occurring 20 minutes prior to sampling. Participants were asked to place a cotton dental swab along their gumline for 30 seconds. The swab was then placed in a syringe and the plunger was depressed to express the saliva into a microcentrifuge tube. The saliva samples were subsequently frozen and sent to Duke University for assaying.

First-day/last-day assessments (longer-term effects)

Range of motion measurements   A goniometer was used for these assessments. This device has two connecting arms with one arm remaining stationary with the proximal part of the joint, whereas the other arm moves with the distal part of the joint to determine the arc of motion that has occurred across the joint. These measures included neck extension and shoulder abduction.

Results

Data analyses suggested that anxiety levels, mood disturbance, neck and shoulder pain and back pain were lower for both groups following the massage and relaxation sessions (Table 6.1). Data analyses on saliva revealed lower cortisol (stress hormone values) for only the massage therapy group after the first and last day's session. Only the massage group improved following the treatment period on neck extension. Data analyses on shoulder abduction suggested that only the massage therapy group improved on this measure by the end of the study (Fig. 6.1).

Table 6.1   Means for massage therapy and relaxation groups for first-/last-day measures

	Massage therapy		Control group	
	First day	Last day	First day	Last day
Neck extension	58^a	66^{bt}	60^a	62^a
Shoulder abduction	148^a	154^{b*}	151^a	148^a

^{a,b}Different letter superscripts indicate significantly different values.
$^*p<0.05$, $^†p<0.01$.

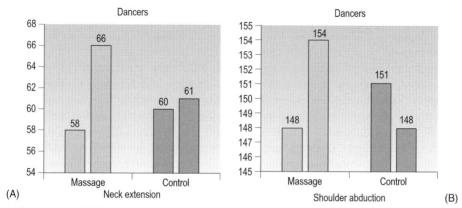

Figure 6.1   (A) Neck extension and (B) shoulder abduction in dancers improved only in the massage therapy group.

Discussion

Only those who received massage therapy showed a decrease in cortisol after the massage treatment. Although decreased anxiety is consistent with the stress reduction literature on massage and relaxation therapies (Field et al 1992, 1996, Platania-Solaazzo et al 1992), a number of studies have shown that massage therapy is more effective than relaxation for reducing stress hormones (Field et al 1992, 1996, Sunshine et al 1996).

The dancers in the present study also reported reduced back, neck and shoulder pain following the massage and relaxation therapy. Similar findings have been reported in other massage therapy studies for chronic pain conditions, including fibromyalgia (Sunshine et al 1996), migraine headaches (Hernandez-Reif et al 1998), lower back pain (Hernandez-Reif et al 2001), and premenstrual syndrome (Hernandez-Reif et al 2000).

In the present study, although both groups reported reduced pain, only the massage therapy group showed improved range of motion (neck extension and shoulder abduction), suggesting that massage therapy may be a more effective treatment for dancers. There are several reasons that might explain why massage therapy effects were superior to relaxation effects for range of motion. First, massage therapy may be stimulating deep pressure receptors, which in turn may be activating parasympathetic activity as evidenced by the reduction in cortisol. This more relaxed state may be more optimal for increasing range of motion. Second, massage therapy works on specific muscles that may be released or loosened with pressure and friction. Perhaps massage therapy stretched the dancers more than relaxation therapy, thus leading to the improved range of motion for the massage therapy group. Finally, it is also possible that the dancers assigned to the relaxation therapy group did not comply with the relaxation sessions, thus obscuring potential effects of relaxation therapy.

STUDY 2: SPINAL CORD PATIENTS BENEFIT FROM MASSAGE THERAPY

The present study assessed massage therapy and exercise effects on C5–C7 spinal cord injury patients (Diego et al 2002). The massage therapy was designed to increase upper body muscle strength and range of motion and improve functionality. Massage therapy has been shown to increase range of motion and reduce pain in lower back pain patients (Hernandez-Reif et al 1998) and in dancers (Leivadi et al 1999) and reduce stiffness, pain, and fatigue in patients with fibromyalgia (Sunshine et al 1996). In addition, massage therapy may reduce the anxiety and depression noted in spinal cord patients (Craig et al 1997, Elliot & Frank 1996, Field 1998). Massage therapy has decreased self-reports of anxiety and depression and has decreased stress hormones (cortisol and norepinephrine) and increased serotonin levels in adults (Field 1998, Hernandez-Reif et al 1998). The exercise routine, although to a lesser degree, was also expected to improve muscle strength, range of motion and functionality and decrease depression and anxiety scores. Exercise has been associated with both physiological and psychological improvements in chronic spinal cord patients. For example, exercise has been associated with improved quality of life scores, cardiovascular, respiratory and muscular activity (Noreau & Shephard 1995).

Method

Subjects

Participants having had spinal cord injuries for at least 1 year were recruited for this study. The study volunteers were first stratified on range of motion and then randomly assigned to either a massage therapy or exercise group.

Interventions

Massage therapy The massage therapy group received a 40-minute massage therapy session twice per week for 5 weeks by trained massage therapists. Participants were massaged on a massage table as follows: arms: (1) moderate pressure and long smooth stroking along the length of each arm, (2) slow stroking with moderate pressure to the muscle attachments at bony landmarks of arms and shoulders, (3) lifting and pulling of the skin along the length of both arms, (4) kneading from shoulder to fingers, (5) applying moderate pressure with both thumbs to spastic areas, (6) carefully stretching the shoulder, elbow, wrist and finger joints; trunk: (1) moderate pressure, long strokes along the length of the back, (2) stroking with moderate pressure to the muscle attachments at bony landmarks of the back, (3) lifting and pulling of the skin along the length of both sides of the spine, (4) kneading the muscles, (5) applying moderate pressure with both thumbs to spastic areas, (6) stretching the back muscles and shoulders, (7) stroking along the entire back and arms.

Exercise treatment   The exercise group was taught an exercise routine that they performed twice per week for 5 weeks on their own. The procedure consisted of slowly repeating the following movements five times (1 minute each):

1. Slowly moving chin to chest and back.
2. Tilting head to each shoulder.
3. With arms by the side raising each shoulder.
4. Raising each arm parallel to ground as high as possible.
5. Extending both arms away from the body at shoulder level and then pulling them back keeping them raised at shoulder level.
6. Interlocking fingers of both hands and then raising both arms, extended, to shoulder level. Then rounding shoulders first in clockwise and then in counterclockwise directions.

The participants were asked to recall each time they conducted this exercise treatment.

Short-term assessments

State Anxiety Inventory (STAI) (Spielberger et al 1970)   This is a 20-item scale that measures the transitory anxiety levels in terms of severity, with 1 = 'not so much' and 4 = 'very much'. Characteristic items include 'I feel tense' and 'I feel relaxed'.

Longer-term assessments

Center for Epidemiological Studies–Depression scale (CES–D) (Radloff 1977)   This is a 20-item questionnaire, with possible scores between 0 and 60. The respondents rate the frequency (within the last week) of 20 symptoms. Symptoms include depressed mood, feelings of helplessness and hopelessness, feelings of guilt and worthlessness, loss of energy, and problems with sleep and appetite.

Manual muscle test   This was used to assess upper limb muscle strength. The Manual Muscle Test was developed to assess motor function after spinal cord injury (Klose et al 1992). Scores for the Manual Muscle Test are as follows: 0 (zero) = no palpable or observable muscle contraction; 1 (trace) = evidence of muscle contraction, no ability to move through the full range of motion (ROM); 2 (poor) = ability to move through the full available ROM (gravity eliminated); 3 (fair) = ability to move through the full available ROM (against gravity); 4 (good) = ability to move through the full available ROM against moderate resistance; and 5 (normal) = ability to move through the full available ROM against maximal resistance.

Range of motion   Range of motion for abduction (shoulders only), extension and flexion of the shoulders, elbows and wrists was assessed by a physical therapist. Range of motion was assessed by placing a goniometer on the axis

Table 6.2   Means for massage and exercise groups before and after massages on the first and last days of the study

	Massage				Exercise			
	First day		Last day		First day		Last day	
	Pre–	Post–	Pre–	Post–	Pre–	Post–	Pre–	Post–
STAI	34.2[a]	25.7[b]	31.6[a]	24.4[b]	31.9[a]	29.2[a]	31.5[a]	29.2[a]
CES-D	15.9[a]		11.4[b]		14.8[a]		15.1[a]	
Muscle strength	4.6[a]		4.8[b]		4.6[a]		4.7[a]	
Range of movement								
Shoulder								
Abduction	125.3[a]		14.37[b]		134.4[a]		141.6[b]	
Flexion	56.4[a]		67.8[a]		69.9[a]		69.1[a]	
Extension	137.0[a]		149.5[a]		154.7[a]		152.2[a]	
Elbow								
Flexion	123.5[a]		135.1[a]		132.7[a]		134.7[a]	
Extension	72.3[a]		83.6[a]		92.2[a]		134.7[a]	
Wrist								
Flexion	63.3[a]		69.5[b]		66.5[ab]		66.9[ab]	
Extension	59.8[a]		66.5[b]		67.4[b]		39.0[b]	

[a,b]Significant differences between numbers.

of the joint and having the therapist help the subject move the extremity through its active range of motion. The greatest angle of motion was then noted in degrees. Range of motion figures for each joint were then averaged for each upper limb yielding seven scores.

Results

The massage group had significantly lower anxiety scores immediately after treatment on the first and last days (see Table 6.2). The massage therapy group experienced a greater decrease in CES-D depression scores. The massage group also showed a greater improvement in muscle strength including shoulder abduction, wrist extension, and wrist flexion (Fig. 6.2).

Discussion

This increased muscle strength and range of motion in the massage group may have contributed to the decrease in their depression and anxiety. Depression is common among patients with spinal cord injury, and is detrimental to their quality of life (Noreau & Shephard 1995). These data suggest that patients with spinal cord injury can benefit from massage therapy. Future studies could assess massage therapy on other spinal cord injury problems including spasticity and pain. Further, other studies are needed to evaluate the effects of massage therapy on the lower extremities of spinal cord injury

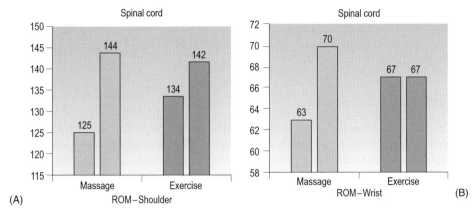

Figure 6.2   The massage group showed a greater improvement in muscle strength: (A) shoulder abduction, (B) wrist extension/flexion.

patients as a means of increasing circulation and minimizing muscle atrophy.

STUDY 3: CEREBRAL PALSY IN CHILDREN DECREASED AFTER MASSAGE THERAPY

The symptoms of cerebral palsy (CP) in children are often severe and wide-ranged including spasticity (rigidity of muscles) and impaired motor organization and functioning (Wiley & Damiano 1998). In addition, children with CP may be cognitively, socially and emotionally impaired (Petersen et al 1998). Massage therapy has been effective for several of the problems related to CP. For example, fine motor functioning, dressing, and arm and leg muscle tone improves following massage therapy in preschool children with Down's syndrome (Hernandez-Reif et al 2005b) and stiffness was reduced in joints of children with chronic juvenile rheumatoid arthritis (Field et al 1997). Massage therapy might also be expected to reduce spasticity, improve muscle tone and range of motion or enhance motor functioning in children with CP. The current study evaluated massage therapy (versus reading as an attention control group) for children with moderate to severe CP for reducing spasticity, improving range of motion, facilitating motor functioning, and enhancing social interactions and development (Hernandez-Reif et al 2005a).

Method

Participants

Twenty preschool children diagnosed with cerebral palsy (CP) participated in this study. Using a random stratification procedure based on age, type of CP (spastic, athetoid, and ataxic) and mobility level (ambulatory, no independent steps, no weightbearing, no sitting), the children were randomly assigned to a massage therapy or a reading attention control group. Spastic cerebral palsy was the most common form of CP, affecting 80% of the participants with the major problems being stiffness and permanently contracted muscles.

Procedure

The children received 30-minute sessions of massage therapy or reading (control group) twice per week for 12 weeks. The one-on-one sessions were conducted in the children's preschool, outside of the classroom in a separate, matted area. The therapist started each session by cradling the child's head and making small circular strokes on the scalp while making eye contact to orient the child to being touched. Subsequently, the therapist applied non-scented oil to his/her hands and massaged the child in the following sequence:

Head/face/scalp:

1. Using flats of fingers, stroking forehead and temple area;
2. Stroking cheekbones outwards toward temple;
3. Massaging, using circular movements, under the chin, cheeks, jawline around the ears, back of neck and base of skull.

Shoulders/arms/hands: applying oil to the hands, then

1. Kneading shoulders, including scapula area, deltoids and pectoral muscles;
2. Making hands like the letter 'C' and milking the arms from the shoulder to the wrist;
3. With hands turning opposite each other, twisting and wringing from the shoulder to the wrist and off the hand;
4. Using thumb-over-thumb motion to massage the palm of the hand;
5. Massaging and gently pulling each finger;
6. Massaging the top of the hand, including the wrist and areas in between fingers;
7. Flexing and extending wrist and fingers;
8. Rolling the arm from shoulder to wrist;
9. Using long milking strokes and smooth strokes from wrist to shoulder.

Chest:

1. Making small finger circles down and then up both sides of sternum;
2. Making small lateral movements with fingertips under clavicles from sternum to shoulder, working both sides of chest simultaneously;
3. With one hand on each shoulder, squeezing whole deltoid area with entire hand, then lightly moving both shoulders back and forth to open up chest area (relaxing and repeating three times).

Hips:

1. Without forcing joints since knees may not bend, holding the lower legs and moving both knees toward chest (relaxing and repeating three times);
2. Repeating same step but alternating lower leg towards opposite shoulder (relaxing and repeating three times).

Legs and feet: applying oil to the hands following procedure for arms and hands to one then the other leg and foot.
Back:

1. Holding chest with fingers and thumbs on child's back, applying small thumb circles down sides of spine from the neck to the tailbone and back up to the neck;
2. Making soothing circular strokes around the tops of the shoulders;
3. Using heel of hand, making circles around entire back, including shoulder blade and lower back areas;
4. Making large full palm circles across entire back.

Reading attention control

The reading sessions were conducted on the same time schedule as the massage sessions. Children in this group were seen twice a week for 12 weeks for individual 30-minute sessions. The sessions were held in the same matted area as the massage. The reading teacher held the child in her lap while reading and showing the child books from the Dr Seuss series. The purpose of this group was to control for potential attention effects that might result from the individual attention therapists were giving the children in the massage therapy group.

Assessments

On the first and last day of the study, the children were assessed prior to massage or reading on the following measures.

Spasticity Scale/Modified Ashworth Scale   This scale ranges from 0 (no increase in muscle tone) to 4 (affected part[s] rigid in flexion or extension). The therapist assessed tone by extending each arm at the shoulder, elbow and wrist separately, over 1 second, and then moving each part to a position of maximal possible flexion for 1 second. The same procedure as conducted for the arms was conducted for the right and left leg, except that extensions and flexions were at the hip, knee and the ankle.

Arms, Legs and Trunk Muscle Tone Scale (ALT Muscle Tone Scale)   This scale was designed for a Down's syndrome massage therapy study (Hernandez-Reif et al 2005b) to assess muscle tone. The scale is rated on a Likert continuum, ranging from 'severe hypertonicity' (4), to 'moderate' (3), to 'mild' (2), to 'slight hypertonicity' (1), to 'normal' (0), to 'slight hypotonicity' (−1), to 'mild' (−2), to 'moderate' (−3), to 'severe hypotonicity' (−4).

Range of motion   Using a goniometer, joint range of motion was measured for hip abduction, aligning the goniometer at the intersection of the hip and thigh joint, moving the thigh away from the hip joint to measure stiffness; and hip extension, placing the child on the right hip and aligning the goniometer on the left hip bone, assessing straightening of the left hip and legs (and repeating on the other hip).

Developmental Measures—Developmental Programming for Infants and Young Children (DPIYC) (Rogers & D'Eugenio 1977)   This scale, designed to yield an early intervention developmental profile, includes six subscales: perceptual, fine motor, gross motor, self-care (feeding, toileting, dressing/hygiene skills), social/emotional, language and cognition. Each child's range of functioning is determined following brief observations with and without objects in open-ended activities. When criteria are met (e.g. repeatedly finding toy when hidden under multiple covers), the item receives a pass (P). The child's functioning level is determined by the age range containing the child's highest passed item.

Results

Data analyses revealed, for the massage therapy group, reduced arm spasticity, improved muscle tone for overall body and arms, and improved right hip and leg extension (see Table 6.3). Data analyses also suggested that the massage therapy group showed improved cognition, fine motor, gross motor, dressing and social functioning. The reading control group had improved language and feeding (see Table 6.4).

Discussion

A reduction in spasticity is optimal, as spastic tone disorder leads to increased muscle tone or rigidity, decreased range of motion and the formation of contractures and limited movement patterns (Harris 1997). In addition, range of motion scores for hip extension improved for the CP children receiving massage therapy, further supporting the finding of overall reduction in hypertonicity (Fig. 6.3). Perhaps the reduced spasticity led to the improved muscle tone or vice versa, and these improvements led to more optimal range of motion. Improved muscle tone findings have also been reported for young children with Down's syndrome receiving massage therapy (Hernandez-Reif et al 2005b).

The children in the massage therapy group showed improved scores in cognition, fine and gross motor functioning, dressing and social skills. Several studies have reported that massage leads to enhanced alertness as measured by EEG (Field 1998) and increases cognitive scores in preschool children (Hart

Table 6.3   Means for massage therapy and reading control group for first versus last day's physical measures

Variables	Massage (N = 10)		Reading control (N = 10)	
	First day	Last day	First day	Last day
Ashworth Spasticity (lower is optimal)				
Arms	2.7^a	1.8^{b*}	2.2^a	2.0^a
Legs	2.3^a	1.8^a	2.0^a	2.2^a
ALT Muscle Tone (4 = hypertonic; 0 = normal; −4 = hypotonic)				
Overall	2.5^a	2.0^{b*}	2.6^a	2.4^a
Arms	2.7^a	2.0^{b*}	2.4^a	2.3^a
Legs	2.4^a	2.1^a	2.6^a	2.1^b
Range of motion				
Hip abduction (higher is optimal)				
Right	27^a	28^a	20^a	18^a
Left	28^a	20^a	18^a	19^a
Hip extension (0 is optimal)				
Right	31^a	11^{b*}	13^a	17^a
Left	25^a	9^{b*}	17^a	13^a

^{a,b}Different letter superscripts reflect significant difference between adjacent means within each group.
*$p<0.05$.

Table 6.4   Means for massage therapy and reading control group for first versus last day for developmental measures

Variables	Massage		Reading control	
	First day	Last day	First day	Last day
Developmental profile (DPIYC) in months (higher is optimal)				
Cognition	7.1^a	8.0^{b*}	10.2^a	10.8^a
Language	9.0^a	10.1^a	10.7^a	11.7^{b*}
Fine motor skills	4.9^a	6.4^{b*}	9.7^a	10.4^{b*}
Gross motor skills	5.8^a	6.8^{b*}	6.0^a	6.2^a
Feed	8.6^a	10.2^a	8.1^a	10.4^{b*}
Toilet	9.9^a	9.0^a	6.0^a	7.3^a
Dress	8.3^a	9.5^{b*}	8.8^a	8.8^a
Social	11.4^a	15.4^{b*}	13.9^a	13.4^a

^{a,b}Different letter superscripts reflect significant difference between adjacent means.
*$p<0.05$.

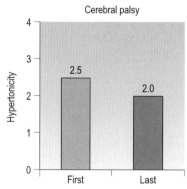

Figure 6.3   Hypertonicity decreased following massage therapy in children with cerebral palsy.

et al 1999) and children with Down's syndrome (Hernandez-Reif et al 2005b).

STUDY 4: CHILDREN WITH DOWN'S SYNDROME IMPROVED IN MOTOR FUNCTION AND MUSCLE TONE FOLLOWING MASSAGE THERAPY

Down's syndrome, a genetic condition affecting 1 in about 700 children born in the United States (Spiker & Hopmann 1997), is characterized by motor development delays (Cadoret & Beuter 1994), and decreased muscle tone or hypotonia (Anneren et al 1996). Because massage therapy has been shown to develop muscle tone for other children (Field 1998), massage therapy might enhance physical development for children with Down's syndrome. If increasing muscle tone facilitates motor functioning, then children with Down's syndrome receiving massage therapy would be expected to show improved motor scores over time. Although no controlled studies were found on massage therapy effects for children with Down's syndrome, one pilot massage study with 13 children with Down's syndrome between 1 and 4 years of age revealed increased muscle activation and less severe hypotonicity (Linkous & Stutts 1990). However, because no comparison group was included in this study, the interpretations are questionable.

The primary objective of the present study was to examine if massage therapy improved muscle tone in children with Down's syndrome and motor development of other areas (Hernandez-Reif et al 2005b). Half of the children with Down's syndrome were assigned to a massage therapy group and the other half to a reading/attention control group. At the beginning and end of a 2-month program (two sessions per week for 8 weeks), muscle tone and development were assessed for the two groups of young children with Down's syndrome. Twenty-three preschool children diagnosed with Down's syndrome were identified for the study.

Method

Procedure

Massage therapy   The same massage procedure as used in the cerebral palsy study (Study 3) above was used here.

Reading attention control   The same reading procedure as used in the cerebral palsy study (Study 3) above was used here.

Assessments

Developmental Programming for Infants and Young Children (DPIYC) (Rogers & D'Eugenio 1977)   This instrument assessed the following areas: perceptual/fine motor, gross motor, self-care (feeding, toileting, dressing/hygiene skills), social/emotional, language and cognition.

Arms, Legs and Trunk Muscle Tone Scale (ALT Muscle Tone Scale) (M Hernandez-Reif & T Field 2000, unpublished work)   The ALT scale was designed during the pilot phase of this study. The ALT ranges along a continuum anchored at one end with a Likert scale for assessing hypotonicity (−4.00 to −1.00), a mid score of 0 to depict normal tone, and anchored at the other end with another Likert scale for assessing hypertonicity (1.00–4.00).

Results

Analyses revealed no group differences on the baseline measures for the DPIYC. Improvement for the reading control group included better scores on gross motor functioning, feeding (self-care), social/emotional functioning, and cognition. The massage therapy group had improved scores on perceptual/fine motor function, gross motor functioning, feeding (self-care), dressing, social/emotional functioning, and cognition (see Table 6.5). Data analyses also revealed an improvement in arm muscle tone for the massage therapy group suggesting less hypotonicity in the arms and legs by the last day of therapy (see Table 6.6; Fig. 6.4).

Discussion

The analyses on change scores revealed developmental gains in motor and muscle tone for the massage therapy group. Increased muscle strength might have contributed to better muscle tone for the massage therapy group from the pressure stimulation. Increasing muscle tone has also been associated with increased functional activity, movement and coordination (Harris 1997) and may explain the improved fine motor and gross functioning scores for

Table 6.5 Mean functioning months for massage therapy and reading/control groups on first and last day's measures

	Massage therapy		Reading/control	
Age (months)	24.4		25.1	
Variables	First day	Last day	First day	Last day
Development (DPIYC)				
Fine motor skills	13.1	18.9	13.1	15.4
Gross motor skills	13.7	24.3	12.3	17.6
Feeding	14.0	19.7	12.2	15.5
Toileting	14.5	17.8	14.9	17.3
Dressing	12.9	20.8	13.1	18.9
Social	18.2	26.5	15.6	20.6
Language	13.1	16.9	11.1	12.5
Cognition	13.8	17.9	12.3	15.7

The first mean for each group represents the baseline developmental age for the group. The second mean for each group represents the developmental age at the end of the study.

Table 6.6 Means for arms, legs and trunk muscle tone for massage therapy and reading control groups

	Massage therapy		Reading/control	
	First day	Last day	First day	Last day
Arms	−2.0	−0.9	−2.5	−3.0
Legs	−2.1	−0.9	−2.3	−2.2
Trunk	−1.8	−0.8	−2.4	−1.3

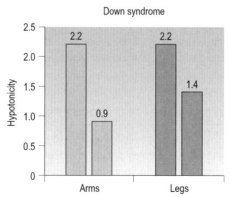

Figure 6.4 Hypotonicity decreased following massage therapy in children with Down's syndrome.

the massage therapy group. The improved muscle tone for the massage therapy children, coupled with their improved motor functioning, is encouraging in that hypotonia (or decreased muscle tone) is common to Down's syndrome and has been related to difficulty in regulating muscle control and stiffness, motor delays and movement patterns (Block 1991).

STUDY 5: PARKINSON'S DISEASE SYMPTOMS ARE REDUCED BY MASSAGE THERAPY

Parkinson's disease affects approximately one in every 100 Americans over the age of 60 (National Institute of Neurological Disorders and Stroke of the National Institutes of Health 2000). Characteristic symptoms include tremors, slowness in executing movements and dopamine deficiency (Lien & Mutch 1997). Other symptoms include impaired daily living activities (Pal et al 2001). Standard medical care includes L-dopa, which increases brain dopamine (Jenner & Brin 1998). Aversive effects of L-dopa include motor fluctuations and dyskinesias (involuntary limb and facial movements) (Jenner & Brin 1998). Alternative therapies may attenuate side-effects without adverse effects of drug therapy, for example, low-frequency muscle stimulation. The present study examined massage therapy as compared to progressive muscle relaxation effects on Parkinson's disease patients (Hernandez-Reif et al 2002).

Method

Participants

Inclusion criteria included:

- age between 50 and 70 years
- <stage 2.5 on the Hoehn–Yahr scale (a disease severity scale from 1 to 5, with 1 = mild and 5 = severe)
- medication stability for the month prior to admission into the study.

Following stratification for disease severity and dyskinesias, 16 participants were randomly assigned to a massage therapy or progressive muscle relaxation group.

Procedure

Massage therapy   Participants in this group received two 30-minute sessions a week for 5 weeks by a trained massage therapist. The massage therapy included the following steps with the patient in the prone position for the first 15 minutes:

- Back: long gliding strokes to the back (2 min); kneading and friction of the shoulder area and upper arms and then general kneading to the back muscles (3 min).

- Buttocks: kneading and pressure to the gluteal muscle area, including applying pressure to specific points where muscle tightness or tender points are noted until the muscles relax (2 min); friction to tight tendons (1 min).
- Ribs: stretching small muscles between the ribs (1 min).
- Thigh: kneading, friction and tendon stretches to the hamstrings (2 min).
- Calf: kneading and friction to the back of the calf with emphasis on the Achilles tendon, attending to tight areas or tender points found (2 min).
- Feet: general kneading of the feet; with the knee slightly bent, flexing the foot toward the back of the calf (2 min).

With participant in the supine position for the final 15 minutes:

- Thigh: friction and pressure to the front, upper thigh area, including applying pressure to specific points where muscle tightness or tender points are noted until muscles relax (2 min); friction to the small muscles focused just above the knee (1 min).
- Lower leg: stretching (longitudinal and transverse) and small finger kneading of the underside of the leg (2 min).
- Feet: kneading the foot followed by flexing the foot to stretch the Achilles tendon (1 min).
- Range of motion: taking each joint (hips, knees, ankles and toes) into flexion and lightly into other ranges of motion (2 min).
- Hands: kneading the hands and fingers (1 min).
- Forearms: kneading and friction to tendons and muscles (1 min).
- Upper arms: kneading and friction to biceps and triceps (2 min).
- Neck: gentle squeezing of muscle immediately inferior to the hairline with moderate pressure, using caution to avoid the major blood vessels (1 min).
- Face: circular finger-tip kneading to the face, especially the forehead, under the eyes (all around the eyes) and around the jaw (1 min).
- Head: scalp kneading (i.e. 'shampooing') (1 min).

Progressive muscle relaxation   The attention control group received progressive muscle relaxation therapy that consisted of the participants lying on their back while listening to a cassette tape leading them through the exercise steps. These 30-minute sessions involved the participant tightening and then relaxing the same large muscle groups that were massaged in the massage group starting at the feet and progressing to the face. The muscle groups that were exercised included the feet, calves, thighs, back, arms (including hands), and face.

Assessments

First–day/last–day measures (long–term effects)   On the first and last day of the study, participants were rated by their physicians, completed self-reports on functioning, sleep and fatigue, and provided a urine sample to assay biochemical levels.

Activities of Daily Life scale (Schwab & England 1958)   This scale rated at 10% increments measures the amount of daily living activities a patient with Parkinson's disease can perform. For example, a score of 100% reflects complete independence and normal performance of chores and a score of 40% identifies a patient who is very dependent, can conduct few chores alone but can assist with all chores.

Sleep scale (Verran & Snyder-Halperin 1988)   Questions on this 15-item scale are rated on a visual analog anchored at one end with effective sleep and at the opposite end with ineffective responses.

Urine samples   Urine samples were collected early in the morning on the first and last days of the study to assess for treatment effects on biochemistry levels. Each sample was frozen and sent to Duke University for analysis.

Results

The physicians rated the massage therapy group as improved on the Activities of Daily Life scale, suggesting greater independence and more normal functioning on chores (Table 6.7; Fig. 6.5). Less sleep disturbance was reported by the massage therapy group for the last day of the study. Reduced norepinephrine (stress hormone) levels ocurred for the massage therapy group.

Discussion

These data are consistent with previous research showing improvement on activities of daily living following massage therapy, for example, for patients with multiple sclerosis (Hernandez-Reif et al 1998a). The massage therapy group reported less sleep disturbance. Improved sleep following massage therapy has been reported in other studies for individuals with fibromyalgia syndrome (Sunshine et al 1996) and migraine headaches (Hernandez-Reif et al 1998). The report of less sleep disturbance by the massage therapy group

Table 6.7   Means for the massage therapy and muscle relaxation groups

Variables	Massage		Relaxation	
	First day	Last day	First day	Last day
Activities of daily life				
Physician rating (%)	87^a	91^b	89^a	87^a
Sleep disturbance	42^a	22^b	34^a	29^a
Norepinephrine (ng/ml)	48^a	25^b	25^b	33^b

[a,b]Different letter superscripts denote differences in means.

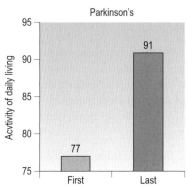

Figure 6.5 Patients with Parkinson's disease showed an improvement in the Activities of Daily Life scale after massage therapy

might have reflected their more relaxed state as evidenced by their decreased urinary norepinephrine (stress hormone) levels at the end of the study. Future research might also consider including a standard care control group and larger sample sizes, as the small sample size for the current study warrants caution in interpreting the findings.

References

Anneren G, Carlsson S, Sara V, et al 1996 The effect of growth hormone therapy on growth and mental development in children with Down syndrome. Developmental Brain Dysfunction 9:138–143.

Block M 1991 Motor development in children with Down syndrome: a review of the literature. Adapted Physical Activity Quaterly 8:179–209.

Cadoret G, Beuter A 1994 Early development of reaching in Down syndrome infants. Early Human Development 36:155–173.

Craig A, Hancock K, Dickson H, et al 1997 Long term psychological outcomes in spinal cord injured persons: results of a controlled trial using cognitive behavior therapy. Archives of Physical Medicine and Rehabilitation 78:33–38.

Diego M, Field T, Hernandez-Reif M, et al 2002 Spinal cord patients benefit from massage therapy. International Journal of Neuroscience 112:133–142.

Elliot T, Frank R 1996 Depression following spinal cord injury. Archives of Physical Medicine and Rehabilitation 77: 816–823.

Field T 1998 Massage therapy effects. American Psychologist 53:1270–1281.

Field T, Morrow C, Valdeon C, et al 1992 Massage therapy reduces anxiety in child and adolescent psychiatric patients. Journal of the American Academy of Child and Adolescent Psychiatry 31:125–131.

Field T, Grizzle N, Scafidi F, et al 1996 Massage and relaxation therapies' effects on depressed adolescent mothers. Adolescence 31:903–911.

Field T, Hernandez-Reif M, Seligman S, et al 1997 Juvenile rheumatoid arthritis: benefits from massage therapy. Journal of Pediatric Psychology 22:607–617.

Harris S 1997 The effectiveness of early intervention for children with cerebral palsy and related motor disabilities. In: Guralnick MJ (ed.) The effectiveness of early intervention. Paul Brookes Publishing Co., Maryland, pp. 327–347.

Hart S, Field T, Hernandez-Reif M, et al 1998 Preschoolers' cognitive performance improves following massage therapy. Early Child Development and Care 143:59–64.

Hernandez-Reif M, Dieter J, Field T, et al 1998a Migraine headaches are reduced by massage therapy. International Journal of Neuroscience 96:1–11.

Hernandez-Reif M, Martinez A, Field T, et al 2000 Premenstrual symptoms are relieved by massage therapy. Journal of Psychosomatic Obstetrics and Gynaecology 21:9–15.

Hernandez-Reif M, Field T, Krasnegor J, et al 2001 Lower back pain is reduced and range of motion increased after massage therapy. International Journal of Neuroscience 106:131–145.

Hernandez-Reif M, Field T, Largie S, et al 2002 Parkinson's disease symptoms are differentially affected by massage therapy vs. progressive muscle relaxation: a pilot study. Journal of Bodywork and Movement Therapies 6(3):177–182.

Hernandez-Reif M, Field T, Largie S, et al 2005a Cerebral palsy symptoms in children decreased following massage therapy. Early Child Development and Care.

Hernandez-Reif M, Field T, Largie S, et al 2005b Children with Down syndrome improved in motor function and muscle tone following massage therapy. Early Child Development and Care.

Hertz G, Fast A, Feinsilver S, et al 1992 Sleep in normal late pregnancy. Sleep 15:246–251.

Jenner P, Brin M 1998 Levodopa neuorotoxicty: experimental studies versus clinical relevance. Neurology 50:39–48.

Klose K, Needham B, Schmidt D, et al 1992 An assessment of the contribution of electromyographic biofeedback as an adjunct therapy in the physical training of spinal cord injured persons. Archives of Physical Medicine and Rehabilitation 74:453–456.

Leivadi S, Hernandez-Reif M, Field T, et al 1999 Massage therapy and relaxation effects on university dance students. Journal of Dance Medicine & Science 3:108–112.

Lien C, Mutch W 1997 The treatment of Parkinson's disease in older people. Scottish Medical Journal 194:147–150.

Linkous L, Stutts R 1990. Passive tactile stimulation effects on the muscle tone of hypotonic, developmentally delayed young children. Perceptual Motor Skills 71:951–954.

McNair D, Lorr M, Droppleman L 1971 POMS—Profile of Mood States. Educational and Industrial Testing Service, San Diego, CA.

National Institute of Neurological Disorders and Stroke of the National Institutes of Health 2000 Parkinson's disease: hope through research. NIH Publication, June.

Noreau L, Shephard R 1995 Spinal cord injury, exercise and quality of life. Sports Medicine 20: 226–250.

O'Rourke M 1998 Massage therapy in dance medicine. Medical Problems of Performing Artists 13:61–65.

Pal S, Bhattacharya K, Agapito C, et al 2001 A study of excessive daytime sleepiness and its clinical significance in three groups of Parkinson's disease patients taking pramipexole, cabergoline and levodopa mono and combination therapy. Journal of Neural Trasmission 108:71–77.

Petersen M, Kube D, Palmer F 1998 The prevalence and correlates of specific learning difficulties in a representative sample of children with hemiplegia. British Journal of Educational Psychology 5:39–51.

Platania-Solaazzo A, Field T, Blank J, et al 1992 Relaxation therapy reduces anxiety in child/adolescent psychiatry patients. Acta Paedopsychiatrica 55:115–120.

Radloff L 1977 The CES-D scale: a self-report depression scale for research in the general population. Applied Psychological Measurement 1:385–401.

Rogers S, D'Eugenio D 1977 Children with autism. In: Schafer D, Moersch M (eds) Developmental programming for infants and young children, 2nd edn. University of Michigan Press, Ann Arbor, pp 107–121.

Schwab R, England A 1958 Parkinson's disease. Journal of Chronic Diseases 8:488.

Smith R, Cubis J, Brinsmead M, et al 1990 Mood changes, obstetric experience and alterations in plasma cortisol, beta-endorphin and corticotrophin releasing hormone during pregnancy and the puerperium. Journal of Psychosomatic Research 34:53–69.

Spielberger C, Gorsuch R, Lushene R 1970 The State Trait Anxiety Inventory. Consulting Psychologists Press, Palo Alto, CA.

Spiker D, Hopmann M 1997 The effectiveness of early intervention for children with Down Syndrome. In: Guralnick ME (ed.) The effectiveness of early intervention. Academic Press, New York, pp 271–305.

Stikeleather J 1991 Effects of positional release on cervical range of motion. Presented at the 11th International Congress of the World Confederation for Physical Therapy, London.

Sunshine W, Field T, Quintino O, et al 1996 Fibromyalgia benefits from massage therapy and transcutaneous electrical stimulation. Clinical Rheumatology 2:18–22.

Twomey L 1992 A rationale for the treatment of back pain and joint pain by manual therapy. Physical Therapy 72:885–892.

Verran J, Snyder-Halperin R 1988 Do patients sleep in the hospital? Applied Nursing Research 1:95.

Wiley M, Damiano D 1998 Lower-extremity strength profiles in spastic cerebral palsy. Developmental Medicine and Child Neurology 40:100–107.

Chapter 7

Movement studies

Movement through space may have effects that are similar to those of massage therapy, inasmuch as movement also provides moderate-pressure stimulation. For example, as individuals move across the floor, they are receiving pressure stimulation on their feet. In these studies, movement of the limbs and the body through space achieved very similar effects to massage therapy. In a study on children with autism, movement therapy led to increased time on-task in the classroom (Escalona et al 2001). In our study on adolescents with ADHD, movement associated with Tai Chi led to similar improvements and/or a similar increase in time on-task in the classroom (Hernandez-Reif et al 2001). The adolescents showed enhanced attentiveness, which may be required by concentration on Tai Chi movements. They also showed a decrease in hyperactivity, even though they were moving through space. In a study on patients with fibromyalgia, we used a different form of movement therapy, called Eutony (Field et al 2003). In this therapy, several forms of pressure stimulation are experienced, including rubbing the arms with two-foot-long half-inch dowels as in 'rubbing the bones' or rubbing the face with a tennis ball. Eutony sessions also include moving in space, typically with a partner, and, often with the eyes closed. Following this form of therapy, fibromyalgia patients who are usually very sensitive to even light touch, were able to 'rub their bones' with dowels and decrease the high levels of pain they normally experienced. In another study using Tai Chi, senior citizens were able to increase their balance and improve their posture following a series of Tai-Chi-like movement sessions.

STUDY 1: CREATIVE MOVEMENT THERAPY BENEFITS CHILDREN WITH AUTISM

Massage therapy is an effective intervention for children with autism. When given twice a week for a month either by massage therapists (Field et al 1997) or by parents (Escalona et al 2001), massage therapy increased attentiveness and social-relatedness within the classroom and reduced touch aversion. The study using parents as therapists also found that the massage therapy reduced sleep problems, including fussing/crying, self-stimulating behaviors, and night-wakings (Escalona et al 2001).

Only anecdotal reports appear in the literature on movement therapy. However, movement, by virtue of stimulating pressure receptors as the body moves through space, might be expected to result in effects similar to those of massage therapy (Field et al 1997). During massage therapy, stimulation of pressure receptors enhances parasympathetic activity, which slows physiology, reduces stress, and enhances attentiveness (Field et al 1998). Therefore, in the present study, movement therapy was expected to increase attentive behavior including on-task behavior (actively engaging or passively watching), and social relatedness (Hartshorn et al 2001). In addition, the movement therapy was expected to decrease stress behaviors including stereotypes, negative responding to touch and resisting the teacher.

Method

Participants

Thirty-eight 5-year-old children from a school for children with autism were observed during two movement sessions at the beginning and the end of a 2-month period of biweekly sessions. The group sizes ranged from three to eight children. Because a random group assignment could not be performed blindly (the teachers and parents remaining naïve to group assignment), a second cohort of 38 children with autism was observed during two movement therapy classes at the beginning and end of a 2-month period.

Procedure

The 30-minute movement sessions were held twice per week, and the children's behaviors were coded during the first and last movement sessions.

Each child was observed for a total of six 1-minute randomly distributed periods over the first 18 minutes of the movement sessions in order to have an equal number of observations for each child, and in order to evenly observe children across the different movement activities. During each 1-minute time sample unit the behaviors that occurred were checked on a time sample unit sheet. They were then tallied and the percent time each behavior occurred was calculated. The following behaviors were recorded: stereotypical behavior, wandering, responding to touch in a negative manner, on-task active behavior, on-task passive behavior, making eye contact, social-relatedness directed toward the teacher, and resisting the teacher.

Movement therapy sessions   The sessions were given by trained movement therapists. The number of movement activities per session varied from three to five (each approximately 6–10 minutes). The sessions all began with a 'warm-up' activity and ended with a 'cool-down' activity. The 'warm-up' activity was the therapist saying hello to each member of the group and clapping the syllables of each person's name as she greeted that member. The 'cool-down' end of session activity was a song with a specific pattern of movements that did not change. The intermediary activities for each session involved using hoops; jumping in and out of them, putting different body parts in and out of the hoops, following the therapist through an obstacle course of gym mats of different shapes and heights, and moving in time to a tambourine and stopping when the tambourine stopped. An assistant teacher from the children's classroom was present to assist the movement therapist. Children had to remain in specific locations of the room indicated by stickers of footprints on the floor when they were not moving around the room.

Results

By the end of the 2 months the movement therapy children versus the control children were spending less time wandering, less time negatively responding to touch, less time resisting the teacher, and more time showing on-task passive behavior (see Table 7.1).

Discussion

The movement therapy sessions led to an increase in socially-appropriate behaviors and a decrease in socially inappropriate behaviors. The increased on-task behavior is consistent with greater attentiveness to tasks following massage therapy (Field et al 1997, 1998). Further research might explore a common mechanism underlying the effects of these two therapies. For example, the changes in EEG in the direction of heightened alertness following massage therapy (Field et al 1996a) and the increased serotonin levels following massage therapy (Field et al 1996b) and following exercise (Nash 1996) might be contributing factors.

Table 7.1   Mean percent time behavior observed during the first and last days of movement classes for preschoolers with autism

	First day		Last day	
Behavior	Movement	Control	Movement	Control
Stereotypical behaviors	2	3	2	4
Wandering	14	16	10	15
Responding to touch negatively	5	4	1	3
On-task	16	15	37	19
Resisting teacher	9	12	4	10

STUDY 2: ATTENTION DEFICIT HYPERACTIVITY DISORDER: BENEFITS FROM TAI CHI

Attention deficit hyperactivity disorder (ADHD) is characterized by cognitive and behavioral deficits including inattention, impulsivity and hyperactivity. Short-term improvements have been reported in behavioral, academic and social functioning with drug therapy such as methylphenidate hydrochloride (Ritalin). Side-effects make this treatment controversial (Parraga & Cochran 1992). Massage therapy has been effective in increasing time spent on task, reducing fidgeting, improving mood, and lowering hyperactivity scores in adolescents with ADHD (Field et al 1998). Tai Chi might be an alternative non-pharmacological therapy for ADHD children because of its documented health benefits for older age groups. Tai Chi reduces symptoms associated with stress (Jin 1989) and improves mood (Brown et al 1995). The present study examined the effects of Tai Chi on anxiety, mood, hyperactivity and conduct in children with ADHD (Hernandez-Reif et al 2001).

Method

Participants

Thirteen adolescents with a mean age of 14.5 years, with a DSM-IV diagnosis of ADHD, were recruited from a remedial school for adolescents with developmental problems.

Procedure

The design consisted of a baseline phase without Tai Chi, a 5-week Tai Chi phase, and a 2-week follow-up phase without Tai Chi. The teachers were asked to complete the Conners Teacher Rating Scale three times.

Tai Chi   The adolescents were taught Tai Chi postures twice a week over 5 weeks. Each class was 30 minutes long and occurred mid-afternoon. Each session began with slow raising and lowering of the arms in synchrony with breathing exercises for 5 minutes. The adolescents were then taught to perform slow turning and twisting movements of the arms and legs, shifting body weight from one leg to the other, rotating from side to side and changing directions in a sequence of Tai Chi forms.

Results

T-tests suggested the following baseline to Tai Chi therapy changes from teacher ratings: during Tai Chi the children displayed less anxiety, improved conduct (Fig. 7.1), less daydreaming, fewer inappropriate emotions, and less hyperactivity (Table 7.2).

Discussion

These improved scores persisted over the 2-week follow up (no Tai Chi period). These positive effects of Tai Chi on adolescents with ADHD parallel the effects reported for adults including reduced mental and emotional stress (Jin 1992) and improved mood (Jin 1989). Future studies might also compare Tai Chi and massage therapy effects on the reduction of stress hormones

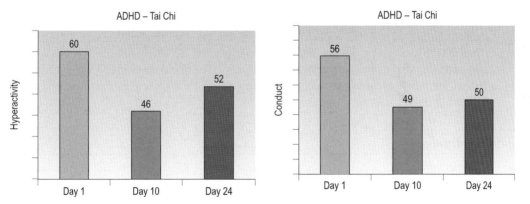

Figure 7.1   Children with ADHD showed improved conduct following Tai Chi.

Table 7.2   Means (and standard deviations in parentheses) on Conners Teacher Rating Scale for baseline, Tai Chi period and 2-week follow-up period.

Variables	Baseline First day	Tai Chi Last day	No Tai Chi (2 weeks later)	F	p value
Conners anxiety	56.7 (11.3)[a]	43.5 (9.6)[b]	44.5 (6.3)[b]	11.9	0.000
Asocial	52.3 (15.2)[a]	46.5 (9.7)[a]	48.7 (10.9)[a]	1.4	0.262
Conduct	56.2 (8.0)[a]	49.0 (11.8)[b]	50.5 (11.9)[b]	5.2	0.013
Daydream	61.0 (6.4)[a]	48.4 (11.6)[b]	50.5 (7.0)[b]	13.8	0.000
Emotion	60.4 (8.9)[a]	50.2 (13.5)[b]	52.0 (12.3)[b]	9.04	0.001
Hyperactive	60.1 (7.9)[a]	45.8 (10.1)[b]	51.7 (8.2)[b]	23.3	0.000
Total hyperactivity	81.5 (11.6)[a]	58.6 (17.8)[b]	66.2 (13.9)	19.49	0.000

[a,b]Different letter superscripts indicate different means.

(e.g. salivary cortisol or urinary catecholamines) in adolescents with ADHD. In addition to few or no side-effects, especially appealing are documented effects of Tai Chi and massage therapy for reducing anxiety and hyperactivity, the major and most difficult symptoms to manage in children with ADHD.

STUDY 3: MOVEMENT AND MASSAGE THERAPY REDUCE FIBROMYALGIA PAIN

Research on exercise suggests that moderate/high intensity exercise has been effective in decreasing fibromyalgia symptoms (Hadhazy et al 2000). In the current study an attempt was made to combine exercise movements with massage therapy to determine whether the combination resulted in greater effects. In addition, the therapy was self-administered. A new field called Eutony, which has been increasingly popular in Europe (most particularly in Germany and France), combines movement and massage therapy techniques that are largely self-administered. The movement part of the Eutony sessions involves stretching movements on the floor and stretching movements through space in an upright position. The self-administered massage involves the rolling of wooden dowels across limbs and the use of balls (e.g. tennis balls) that are again rolled across the surface of the limbs. Pain is noted to diminish following the application of pressure as, for example, in squeezing one's elbow after bumping it and reducing pain. In the present study we hypothesized that the self-administered pressure stimulation involved in the movement and massage aspects of Eutony might be effective in fibromyalgia (Field et al 2003).

Method

Participants

Forty patients with fibromyalgia were recruited from community pain clinics and were randomly assigned to a movement/massage therapy group or a relaxation control group. The participants had spent on average 8.4 years in treatment.

Procedure

Movement/massage therapy   The participants engaged in movements in lying, seated and standing positions (much as in yoga stretching classes). During these stretching exercises they received self-stimulation of pressure receptors by rubbing limbs against the floor and against other limbs. Self-massage was administered using 2-foot-long, 1-inch-diameter wooden dowels and tennis balls. The participants were asked to rub their upper and lower limbs with the wooden dowels, and to rub a tennis ball in a circular fashion on the face, shoulders, arms and hands. The sessions lasted 50 minutes and were held twice per week for 3 weeks.

Progressive muscle relaxation therapy   A relaxation group was assessed to control for potential placebo effects or improvement related to the increased attention given to the massage therapy group participants. The relaxation therapy group was given instructions on how to conduct progressive muscle relaxation sessions for 50 minutes while lying quietly on a carpeted floor (similar floor as the movement/massage therapy group used). The muscle relaxation included tensing and relaxing large muscle groups starting with the head and moving to the neck, shoulders, back, arms, hands, legs, and feet. The therapist conducted these sessions twice a week for 3 weeks.

Assessments

The questionnaires and assessments were given pre- and post-sessions on the first and last days of the study to measure the effects of the therapy in the following order:

1. The State Anxiety Inventory (STAI; Spielberger et al 1970)
2. The Profile of Mood States (POMS; McNair et al 1971)
3. The Regional Pain Scale—a drawing of 21 regions on the front and back of the body where pain is to be rated.

Results

As can be seen in Table 7.3, both groups showed decreased anxiety and pain after the first and/or last sessions. However, only the movement massage therapy group experienced improved mood, lower anxiety and less pain (Fig. 7.2) across the course of the study.

Discussion

The movement/massage therapy patients' reports of less depressed mood, anxiety and pain across the study were consistent with our previous findings on massage therapy effects with fibromyalgia (Sunshine et al 1996). The data from the current study, however, suggested that massage-like stimulation can be self-administered and still result in reduced pain.

Table 7.3   Means for effects of movement/massage therapy

| | Relaxation | | | | Movement/massage | | | |
| | First session | | Last session | | First session | | Last session | |
Variables	Pre–	Post–	Pre–	Post–	Pre–	Post–	Pre–	Post–
Mood	13	11	15	13	15	8[a]	15	4[a]
Anxiety	55	48[a]	49	49	51	32[a]	35[b]	28[a]
Pain	50	46	46	38[a]	43	32[a]	25[b]	19[a]

[a]Significant pre-/post- differences; [b]significant first/last session differences.

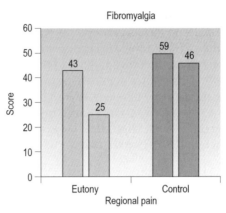

Figure 7.2 Regional pain improved in patients with fibromyalgia following massage therapy. This improvement was greater than in control subjects given relaxation therapy.

STUDY 4: SENIOR CITIZENS BENEFIT FROM MOVEMENT THERAPY

Senior citizens are noted to experience chronic pain (Klinger & Spaulding 1998). Pain management for them is difficult because of side-effects from medications, slower drug metabolism and changes in their cardiovascular and respiratory systems (Richardson & Bresland 1998). Because they have little pain relief and have experienced side-effects of medications, senior citizens are turning to alternative treatments for their pain conditions (Berman & Swyers 1997).

Other problems experienced by this age group include their loss of lower-extremity strength, their unstable gait and a frequent occurrence of falling (Tse & Bailey 1998). Their balance has been improved by Tai Chi (Tse & Bailey 1998). These improvements in balance may have derived from improved muscle strength. The increase in muscle strength and balance may have in turn led to the fewer falls reported following Tai Chi (Province et al 1995).

The purpose of the current study was to try a different type of movement therapy with senior citizens, namely a more creative, larger movement-in-space therapy (Hartshorn et al 2001). The effects of this therapy were assessed by the balance and gait evaluations and by the participants' self-reports on their mood states (depression, anger and vigor) and their pain and strength ratings including overall body pain, back pain and leg pain.

Method

Participants

Thirty-two senior citizens (26 females; mean age = 86 years) were recruited by the activity directors of two retirement communities. They were then randomly assigned to a movement therapy or a wait list control group who were given the movement therapy only after the end of the study. A trained movement therapist led the senior citizens in four 50-minute movement therapy sessions over a 2-week period.

Assessments

The following assessments were collected before the movement therapy or control sessions on the first and last days of the study.

The Profile of Mood States (POMS) (McNair et al 1971)   The participants were asked to indicate how well an adjective (e.g. unhappy, hopeless, guilty) described their current mood state.

Pain and strength ratings   Overall body pain, back pain, and leg pain were rated on visual analog scales (VITAS Healthcare Corporation, FL, USA) ranging from 0 (no pain) to 10 (worst possible pain), anchored with five faces at two-point intervals. Leg strength was rated on a 10-point scale ranging from very weak (0) to moderate (5) to very strong (10).

Tinetti Balance and Gait Evaluation   The Tinetti Balance and Gait Evaluation was used to assess motion in the participants. The balance scale includes items like sitting balance, rising and standing balance, turning 360°, and sitting down. The gait scale includes step length and height (clearing the floor), step continuity, step symmetry, and walking stance.

Movement therapy sessions

The movement therapy sessions lasted 50 minutes each, scheduled over a 2-week period. Music was played in the background for the session. Props were used for the participants to rub themselves on different body parts, for example, rolling a 1-inch diameter yard-long wooden dowel under their feet, down their back or across their thighs for 1-minute periods each. The purpose of this was to stimulate deep pressure receptors, which has been notably effective in massage therapy. The sessions consisted of the following stages:

1. Warm up. This was done while seated in chairs in a circle. Introductions were done verbally and through movement (such as passing around the circle a movement for everyone to mimic), focusing on breathing (breathing deeply together) and doing gentle movements with all body parts such as raising the arms and legs and rotating the head, to kinesthetically sense the body parts. Self-massage was also used as part of this process.
2. Thematic preparation. Larger, whole-body movements were encouraged such as swaying, pushing, stamping, twisting, turning, stepping, and swinging, so that people stretched and used the space more fully. All participants were encouraged to suggest a movement, which could be followed and shared by everyone in the group.
3. Resting and sharing. This was an opportunity for the participants to rest physically and notice any changes in themselves, such as increased heart rate, expanded respiration, and how their bodies had responded to moving.

Although many shared their feelings of well-being during this segment, these comments were not recorded because of their subjective nature.

4. Developing the theme. This was the time when the group worked more specifically with movements that had emerged during the session. People were encouraged to move more freely, for example, to intensify the movement and feeling of swaying or rocking. Sometimes this process was enhanced by working in pairs and mirroring or providing mutual support. A prop such as a ball or rope helped to enlarge or focus a movement. Breathing, progressive relaxation of all body parts, and the use of imagery and visualization were used.

Results

As can be seen in Table 7.4, the participants improved in their functional motion on the Tinetti scale score and specifically on the Gait scale (Fig. 7.3). Leg strength increased and leg pain was significantly decreased.

Table 7.4   Means for measures taken before the first class and after the last class

Measures	First day		Last day	
	Test	Control	Test	Control
POMS (total)[a]	20.8	19.7	20.3	20.4
Overall pain[a]	3.6	3.5	3.1	3.2
Back pain[a]	3.3	3.9	2.2	3.6
Leg pain[a]	3.1	3.1	1.4	2.9
Leg strength[b]	5.5	4.9	6.3	5.1
Total Tinetti score[b]	17.1	18.0	19.3	18.2
Balance[b]	9.1	9.0	9.9	9.4
Gait[b]	8.0	8.4	9.5	9.1

[a] Lower is optimal; [b] higher is optimal.

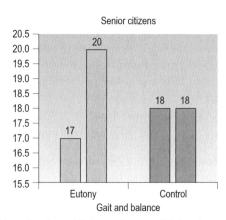

Figure 7.3   Senior citizens' gait and balance improved following movement therapy.

Discussion

The improvement in leg strength probably derived from the leg movements. Strength may have contributed to the improvement in gait including step lengths and height (clearing the floor), step continuity, step symmetry and walking stance. These results are consistent with studies supporting improvements in muscle strength (Lan et al 1998) and in balance (Wolf et al 1997). The freer movements and the lesser degree of structure and concentration required of the elderly may make this a more enjoyable kind of movement therapy than the more frequently studied Tai Chi.

References

Berman B, Swyers J 1997 Establishing a research agenda for investigating alternative medical interventions for chronic pain. Primary Care 24:743–758.

Brown D, Wang Y, Ward A, et al 1995 Chronic psychological effects of exercise and exercise plus cognitive strategies. Medicine, Science and Sports Exercise 27:765–775.

Escalona A, Field T, Singer-Strunk R, et al 2001 Brief report: Improvements in the behavior of children with autism following massage therapy. Journal of Autism and Developmental Disorders 31:513–516.

Field T, Ironson G, Scafidi F, et al 1996a Massage therapy reduces anxiety and enhances EEG pattern of alertness and math computations. International Journal of Neuroscience 86:197–205.

Field T, Grizzle N, Scafidi F, et al 1996b Massage and relaxation therapies effects on depressed adolescent mothers. Adolescence 31:903–911.

Field T, Lasko D, Mundy P, et al 1997 Brief report: Autistic children's attentiveness and responsivity improve after touch therapy. Journal of Autism and Developmental Disorders 27:333–338.

Field T, Quintino O, Hernandez-Reif M 1998 Attention deficit hyperactivity disorder adolescents benefit from massage therapy. Adolescence 33:103–108.

Field T, Delage J, Hernandez-Reif M 2003 Movement and massage therapy reduce fibromyalgia pain. Journal of Bodywork and Movement Therapies 7:49–52.

Hadhazy VA, Ezzo J, Creamer P, et al 2000 Mind–body therapies for the treatment of fibromyalgia: a systematic review. Journal of Rheumatology 27:2911–2918.

Hartshorn K, Delage J, Field T, et al 2001 Senior citizens benefit from movement therapy. Journal of Bodywork and Movement Therapies 5:1–5.

Hernandez-Reif M, Field T, Thimas E 2001 Attention deficit hyperactivity disorder: benefits from Tai Chi. Journal of Bodywork and Movement Therapies 5:120–123.

Jin P 1989 Changes in heart rate, noradrenaline, cortisol and mood during Tai Chi. Journal of Psychosomatic Research 33:197–206.

Jin P 1992 Efficacy of Tai Chi, brisk walking, meditation and reading in reducing mental and emotional stress. Journal of Psychosomatic Research 36:361–370.

Klinger L, Spaulding S 1998 Chronic pain in the elderly: is silence really golden? Physical and Occupational Therapy in Geriatrics 15:1–17.

Lan C, Lai J, Chen S, et al 1998 12-month Tai Chi training in the elderly: its effect on health fitness. Medicine and Science in Sports and Exercise 30:345–351.

McNair D, Lorr M, Droppleman L 1971 Profile of Mood States. Educational and Industrial Testing Services, San Diego.

Nash R 1996 The serotonin connection. Journal of Orthomolecular Medicine 11:327–328.

Parraga HC, Cochran MK 1992 Emergence of motor and vocal tics during imipramine administration in two children. Journal of Child and Adolescent Psychopharmacology 2:227–234.

Province M, Hadley E, Hornbrook M 1995 The effects of exercise on falls in elderly patients. A preplanned meta-analyses of the FICSIT trials. Frailty and Injuries: Cooperative studies on intervention techniques. Journal of American Medical Association 273:1341–1347.

Richardson J, Bresland K 1998 The management of postsurgical pain in the elderly population. Drugs and Aging 13:17–31.

Spielberger CD, Gorsuch RC, Lushene RE 1970 The State Trait Anxiety Inventory. Consulting Psychologists Press, Palo Alto.

Sunshine W, Field TM, Quintino O, et al 1996 Fibromyalgia benefits from massage therapy and transcutaneous electrical stimulation. Journal of Clinical Rheumatology 2:18–22.

Tse S, Bailey D 1998 Tai Chi and postural control in the well elderly. American Journal of Occupational Therapy 46:295–300.

Wolf S, Barnhart H, Ellison G, et al 1997 The effect of Tai Chi Quan and computerized balance training on postural stability in older subjects. Atlanta FICSIT Group. Frailty and injuries. Cooperative studies on intervention techniques. Physical Therapy 77:371–381.

Chapter **8**

Pain reduction

CHAPTER CONTENTS

Massage therapy is most popularly used with pain syndromes. One of the most common mechanisms used to explain massage therapy effects is the gate theory. In this theory, pain is noted to stimulate shorter and less myelinated (or less insulated) nerve fibers so that the pain message takes longer to reach the brain than the pressure message, which is transmitted by nerve fibers that are more insulated and longer and therefore able to transfer the stimulus faster. The message from the pressure stimulation reaches the brain prior to the pain message and, thereby, 'closes the gate' to the pain stimulus. Another theory is that massage therapy enhances deep sleep or restorative sleep. In deep sleep, less substance P is emitted, leading to less pain (given that substance P causes pain). Although the precise mechanism is not yet known, there are several pain syndromes that have benefited from massage therapy. In this chapter, we present data on burn, trauma, back pain, fibromyalgia and carpal tunnel syndrome. In the first study, patients afflicted with burns were noted to have higher thresholds during the painful 'skin brushing' procedure if they were given massage therapy before the procedure (Hernandez-Reif et al 2001). Massage therapy may have led to increased pain thresholds, enabling the patients to endure that procedure with less difficulty. Figure 8.1 shows a proposed model for the symptom-alleviating effects of massage therapy. In another study, patients with low back pain experienced fewer days of low back pain following a period of massage therapy (Hernandez-Reif et al 2000). In our study on patients with fibromyalgia, the 'enhanced deep sleep leading to less substance P' theory was more directly tested (Field et al 2002). In that study, the amount of deep sleep was recorded, and substance P was assayed in saliva samples. Notably, following a period of massage therapy, more time was spent in deep sleep, and lower levels of substance P were noted. In our study on carpal tunnel syndrome, the patients received massage therapy from a therapist once a week and gave themselves the massage the other days of the week (Field et al 2004). Following a period of massage therapy, the nerve conduction velocity or the speed with which electrical stimuli could be transmitted across the neuron was more rapid, suggesting an improvement in the carpal tunnel syndrome condition.

STUDY 1: CHILDREN'S DISTRESS DURING BURN TREATMENT IS REDUCED BY MASSAGE THERAPY

Children less than 4 years old are at greater risk for burn-related deaths since their skin is thin and can be deeply burned at low temperatures. Debridement (skin brushing) and/or dressing-change procedures for treating severe burns can be painful and stressful for young patients. Pain management, such

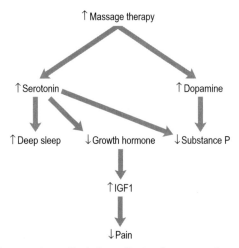

Figure 8.1 Model for symptom-alleviating effects of massage therapy.

as the administration of opioid analgesics, may decrease pain levels, and anxiolytics have been used to reduce anticipatory procedural anxiety. Because side-effects of these medications can lead to respiratory dysfunction (Latarjet & Choinere 1995), complementary treatments are being used for pain management. They may offer a safer approach for reducing pain and procedural anxiety.

In an earlier study we reported that adult burn patients who received daily massage therapy had reduced anxiety and pain, and their cortisol (stress hormone) levels were also lower following massage therapy (Fig. 8.2). Because massage therapy has not been evaluated for reducing procedural anxiety or pain for burned children, the present study examined whether massage therapy could lower burned children's stress behaviors during dressing changes (Hernandez-Reif et al 2001).

Method

Participants

Twenty-four children (mean age = 29.3 months) were enrolled in this study shortly after admission at a burn unit. After informed consent, the children were randomly assigned to a massage therapy (n = 12) or standard care control group (n = 12).

Procedure

Standard medical care   Approximately 30 minutes prior to dressing changes, children were given an analgesic.

Attention control group   To control for attention or placebo effects, the massage therapist spent 15 minutes with the children assigned to the control

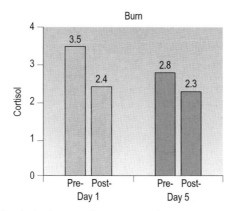

Figure 8.2   Cortisol levels for burn patients pre- and post-massage sessions on day 1 and day 5 of massage therapy study.

group prior to dressing changes. During the 15-minute period, the massage therapist sat next to the child's bed and talked with the child.

Massage therapy   Children assigned to the massage therapy group received a 15-minute massage from a trained therapist prior to dressing changes (Fig. 8.3). The following strokes were applied with moderate pressure to the areas of the child's body that were *not* burned:

Face:

1. Small circles to entire scalp (as if shampooing hair).
2. Using flats of fingers, long stroking to both sides of face.
3. Starting at midline of forehead, stroking with flats of fingers outward towards temples.
4. Small circular stroking over the temples and jaw area.
5. Using flats of fingers, stroking over the nose, cheeks, jaw, and chin.

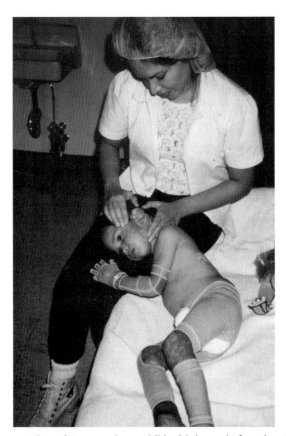

Figure 8.3   Massage therapist massaging a child with burns before dressing changes.

Legs:

1. Three long gliding strokes from the feet to the hips.
2. Squeezing and twisting in wringing motion from the feet to the knees.
3. Gliding thumbs across the bottom of each foot, followed by squeezing and tugging of each toe.
4. Stretching the Achilles tendons by flexing and extending each foot.

Arms:

1. Stroking from hands to shoulders.
2. Same procedure as for legs.

Back and shoulders:

1. Long gliding movements downward along the back from the neck to the hip.
2. Hand-over-hand movements from the upper to the lower back.
3. Starting at the top of the spine, alternating hand strokes across the back working down towards the tail bone (never pressing the spine) and reaching over to include sides.
4. Rubbing and kneading shoulders.
5. Small, circular rubbing along the base of the neck.
6. Long, gliding stroking from the base of the neck and down the length of the back to the tailbone.

Assessments

Behavior observations   Immediately following the intervention, an observer unaware of the child's group assignment (massage versus control), recorded the child's behavior before and during the dressing change. The Children's Hospital of Eastern Ontario Pain Scale (CHEOPS) (McGrath et al 1985) was used to code the distress behaviors during the observations prior to and during the dressing change. Six behaviors were recorded as shown in Table 8.1.

Post-session only assessments

Nurses' rating scale   Nurses who performed the procedure were asked to complete a short questionnaire. Two questions involved the child's stress level at the beginning and end of the procedure, using a 0 (very relaxed) to 5 (very tense) scale. Two additional questions rated the patient's overall pain, using a 0 (low pain) to 5 (high pain) scale, and the difficulty of the procedure, using a 0 (easy) to 5 (difficult) scale. The nurses who conducted the dressing changes were blind to the children's group assignments.

Massage rating scale   The therapists completed this scale immediately after the massage. The therapists rated the children's and their own stress level at

Table 8.1 The Children's Hospital of Eastern Ontario Pain Scale used to code distress behaviors

Cry	
No cry	1
Moaning	2
Crying	2
Screaming	3
Facial	
Smiling	0
Composed	1
Grimace	2
Verbal	
Positive	0
No talking	1
Other complaint	1
Pain complaint	2
Both complaints	2
Torso	
Neutral	1
Shifting	2
Tense	2
Shivering	2
Upright	2
Restrained	2
Touch	
No touching	1
Reaching	2
Touching	2
Grabbing	2
Restrained	2
Legs	
Neutral	1
Squirm/kick	2
Drawn up/tense	2
Standing	2
Restrained	2

the beginning and end of the massage on a Likert scale ranging from 0 (very tense) to 5 (very relaxed). The therapists also rated on a scale of 0 (not well) to 5 (very well) how the massage therapy session went overall. The criterion for this item was based on the child's responsiveness to receiving massage therapy. For example, a score of 5 on this item reflected that the child was very receptive to being touched and cooperated during the massage session.

Results

CHEOPS

Tests revealed that the massage therapy group showed only an increase in torso movements during the dressing changes (see Table 8.2). In contrast, the control group showed an increase in facial grimacing, torso movement, crying, leg movement, and reaching out.

Nurses' rating scales

The nurses reported less difficulty in completing the procedure for the children who received massage therapy prior to the dressing change.

Massage therapists' rating scale

The massage therapists reported that their stress levels were lower after massaging the children and that the children appeared to be more relaxed after the massage therapy.

Discussion

These results and other data show that massage therapy benefits the therapist as well as the receiver of massage (Field et al 1997a). Future research might study the efficacy of teaching parents to massage their children prior to burn care procedures to reduce the anticipatory stress level of both parties. One limitation of our study was the small sample size. Future studies need to be conducted with larger samples. Another future study might assess having the children serve as their own controls to provide a better measure of massage therapy outcome. Assessing neuropeptide pain levels (substance P) during stressful medical procedures could provide additional measures of massage therapy effects as an adjunct to standard burn dressing care.

Table 8.2 Means of Children's Hospital of Eastern Ontario Pain Scale ratings (0–3) of distress behaviors observed before and during dressing change

Variables	Massage therapy		Control	
	Before dressing	During dressing	Before dressing	During dressing
Crying	1.5^a	1.8^a	1.3^a	1.9^b
Facial	1.3^a	1.6^a	1.4^a	1.8^b
Verbal	1.0^a	1.0^a	1.0^a	1.1^a
Torso	1.0^a	1.5^b	1.2^a	1.8^b
Touch	1.1^a	1.1^a	1.0^a	1.4^b
Legs	1.0^a	1.1^a	1.0^a	1.4^b

Lower scores are optimal. ^{a,b}Different superscripts denote differences for adjacent means within groups.

STUDY 2: LOWER BACK PAIN IS REDUCED AND RANGE OF MOTION INCREASED AFTER MASSAGE THERAPY

The morbidity associated with back pain is the most frequent cause of job absenteeism (Courtney & Webster 1999). Pain medications often have side-effects such as drowsiness and impaired cognitive function. Therefore alternatives to medication are attractive for relieving chronic back pain. Relaxation therapy has been used for lower back pain (Nicholas et al 1992) as has massage therapy, but the studies have been methodologically flawed and massage has only been assessed as a control rather than as an intervention (see Ernst 1999). The present study examined massage and relaxation therapy for lower back pain (Hernandez-Reif et al 2001).

Method

Participants

The sample included 24 adults with low back pain. Exclusion criteria were back pain due to fractured vertebrae, herniated or degenerated disks, patients who had undergone surgery for their back pain and patients with sciatic nerve involvement. Participants were randomly assigned to a massage therapy or relaxation therapy group.

Procedure

Massage therapy   The massage consisted of the following techniques applied to the entire back at a level tolerant to the subject:

1. Moving the flats of the hands across the back.
2. Kneading and pressing of muscles.
3. Short back-and-forth rubbing movements to the muscles next to the spine and later to the hip bone (Fig. 8.4).

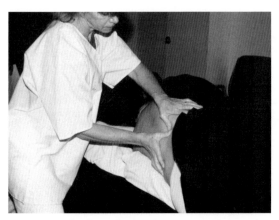

Figure 8.4   Massage therapy for lower back pain.

The following techniques were administered to the legs:

1. Long gliding strokes to the entire leg.
2. Kneading and moving the skin in the thigh area.
3. Pressing and releasing, and back-and-forth rubbing movements to the area between the hip and the knee.
4. Short rubbing movements to the small muscles around the knees.

In the supine position with a bolster under the knee, subjects received:

1. Long gliding strokes and kneading of the neck muscles.
2. Moving the flats of the hands across the abdomen.
3. Pinching and moving the skin on the abdomen in all directions.
4. Kneading the muscles that bend the trunk forward.

Then, to the entire leg:

1. Stroking.
2. Kneading followed by pressing and releasing the anterior thigh region.
3. Slow flexing of the thigh and knee.
4. Slow pulling of both legs.

Relaxation therapy   A relaxation therapy group was included to control for potential placebo effects and the effects of increased attention given to the massage subjects. The relaxation therapy group was given instructions on progressive muscle relaxation exercises, tensing and relaxing large muscle groups starting with the feet and progressing to the calves, thighs, hands, arms, back and face. The subjects were asked to conduct these 30-minute sessions at home twice a week for 5 weeks and to keep a log. Participants also received weekly calls to monitor compliance.

Assessments

Pre-/post-session assessments (immediate effects)   The following assessments were made before and after the sessions on the first and last days of the 5-week study. These measures were used to assess stress, pain and range of motion.

Profile of Mood States Depression scale (POMS-D) (McNair et al 1971)   The POMS consists of 19 adjectives rating depressed mood 'right now' on a five-point scale ranging from 'not at all' to 'extremely' using words such as 'blue', 'sad', and 'lively'.

State Anxiety Inventory (STAI) (Spielberger et al 1970)   The STAI was administered to determine anxiety levels. The STAI is comprised of 20 items and assesses how the subject feels at that moment in terms of severity (not at all to very much so). Characteristic items include 'I feel nervous' and 'I feel calm'.

VITAS (VITAS Healthcare Corporation, FL, USA)   Present pain was also determined with a Visual Analog Scale ranging from 0 ('happy face) to 10 ('frowning/sad face'). This scale included ratings from no pain to worst possible pain.

Range of motion (ROM) measures

While standing, a baseline measure was taken of the length of the spine using a tape measure. Using indelible ink, one mark was made on the skin at the most prominent bone at the base of the neck (cervical vertebra bone 7) and a second mark was made on the skin at the round bony prominence of the backbone (lumbar vertebra 1). The distance between these two marks was recorded in centimeters, with the subject standing with feet shoulder width apart in a normal position. A trunk flexion ROM measure (touch toes without pain) was subsequently recorded, again from the base of the neck (cervical vertebra bone 7) to the round bony prominence of the backbone (lumbar vertebra 1) by asking the subject to reach forward to touch toes without causing pain. The difference between the standing baseline measure and trunk flexion measure served as the trunk flexion ROM. A pain flexion ROM measure (touch toes with pain) was then obtained as above but the subject was asked to reach toward toes or flex the trunk as far as possible, even with pain. This measure was subtracted from the baseline measure.

First–/last–day sessions (longer–term effects)   On the first and last day of the 5-week study, the following assessments were conducted.

Sleep scale (Verran & Snyder-Halperin 1988)   Questions on this 15-item scale are rated on a visual analog anchored at one end with effective sleep responses (e.g. 'Did not awaken', 'Had no trouble sleeping') and at the opposite end with ineffective responses (e.g. 'Was awake 10 hours', 'Had a lot of trouble falling asleep'). Subjects placed a mark across the answer line at the point that best reflected their last night's sleep. The scale yields subcategories of sleep disturbance ('I had a lot of trouble with disrupted sleep'), sleep effectiveness ('Awoke refreshed') and supplementary sleep ('After morning awakening, stayed awake'). A reliability coefficient of 0.82 has been reported for this scale (Snyder-Halperin & Verran 1987).

Urine samples   These were collected on the first and last days of the study and assayed for dopamine and serotonin (5-HIAA) levels. Dopamine and serotonin levels (which may be depleted with chronic pain) were expected to increase in the massage group by the end of the 5-week treatment based on previous literature (Field et al 1996).

Results

Data analyses revealed a greater improvement in mood for the massage group. A decrease in anxiety occurred for both groups after treatment sessions on both days. An effect on the VITAS suggested that only the massage therapy group experienced less pain immediately after their first and last treatment session (Fig. 8.5). Trunk flexion improved for the massage group but only on the first day. The massage therapy group reported less sleep disturbance by the end of the study (Fig. 8.6). Improved range of motion was also noted for the massage therapy group from the first to the last day of the study (Fig. 8.7). Finally, significant increases in serotonin and dopamine occurred, but only for the massage therapy group (Table 8.3).

Discussion

These findings concur with other massage studies on depressive pain syndromes including fibromylagia (Sunshine et al 1996) and chronic fatigue syndrome (Field et al 1997b) and suggest that massage therapy is more effective than relaxation therapy for reducing pain and anxiety and improving mood. The massage therapy group also experienced immediate changes in

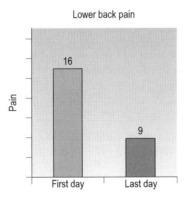

Figure 8.5   Lower back pain rating on first day and last day of massage therapy study.

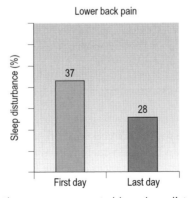

Figure 8.6   The massage therapy group reported less sleep disturbance by the end of the study.

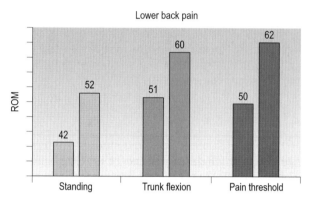

Figure 8.7 Improved range of motion was noted for the massage therapy group from the first to the last day of the study.

Table 8.3 Means for pre-/post-session measures for the massage and relaxation groups

Measures	Massage therapy				Relaxation			
	First day		Last day		First day		Last day	
	Pre-	Post-	Pre-	Post-	Pre-	Post-	Pre-	Post-
Mood (POMS)	14[a]	6[b]	7[b]	7[b]	7[a]	6	1[a]	6[b]
Anxiety (STAI)	36[a]	26[b]	33[a]	28[b]	34[a]	29[b]	33[a]	26[b]
Pain (VITAS)	6[a]	3	4	1[b]	5[a]	4	3[a]	3[b]
Trunk flexion[c] (touch toes without pain)	56[a]	61[b]	59[b]	61[b]	58[a]	58	57[a]	58[a]
Pain flexion[c] (touch toes with pain)	58[a]	60[a]	60[b]	61[b]	61[a]	61	60[a]	61[a]
Sleep disturbance	35[a]		28[b]		32[a]		30[a]	
Dopamine (ng/ml)[c]	209[a]		264[b]		237[a]		195[a]	
Serotonin (ng/ml)[a]	2281[a]		4621[b]		2323[a]		2404[a]	

[a,b]Different letter superscripts indicate different means. [c]Higher score is optimal.

trunk flexion and displayed improved trunk flexion across the study period. Increased range of motion has been correlated with significant pain reduction following physical therapy (Mooney et al 1996). Other effects for the massage therapy group included lower depression scores and less disturbed sleep by the end of the study. Similar findings are reported for other pain syndromes following massage (Field et al 1997c, Sunshine et al 1996,). The increase in serotonin levels for the massage therapy group is encouraging in that serotonin levels may become depleted in individuals with chronic pain (Jhingran et al 1996, Solomon et al 1995). The increase in dopamine values may also be related to the improved mood and pain reduction. Data from animal studies reveal increases in dopamine concentration as a result of circulating opiates (Bergstrom et al 1998).

Future studies might examine sleep recordings and biochemical assays of substance P. Lower back pain may be related to less sleep and the resultant release of substance P, as has been implicated in studies on other pain syndromes (Field et al 2003, Sunshine et al 1996).

STUDY 3: FIBROMYALGIA PAIN AND SUBSTANCE P DECREASE AND SLEEP IMPROVES AFTER MASSAGE THERAPY

Fibromyalgia syndrome (FMS), which affects mostly women, is defined as widespread chronic musculoskeletal pain of unknown etiology and multiple tender points (Russell et al 1994). Substance P levels are significantly elevated (Moldofsky 1993, Russell et al 1994), and low serotonin levels may lead to deep sleep disturbance as well as lower pain thresholds and elevated substance P levels (Juhl 1998, Moldofsky 1993). Antidepressants have been useful for increasing serotonin levels and in turn reducing fibromyalgia symptoms (Russell et al 1992). Non-medical treatments such as relaxation therapy (Beckelew et al 1998), and acupuncture (Berman et al 2000) have also proven promising. We studied massage therapy effects on pain reduction and diminishing sleeping problems in fibromyalgia (Sunshine et al 1996).

In our study, 30 adult FMS patients were randomly assigned to a massage therapy group, a transcutaneous electrical stimulation group, or a no-current transcutaneous electrical stimulation group for 30-minute treatment sessions twice weekly for 5 weeks (Field et al 2002). The massage therapy participants reported lower anxiety and depression, and their cortisol levels were lower immediately after the therapy sessions on the first and last days of the study. By the end of the study, the massage therapy group had improved on the dolorimeter measure of pain. At that time, they also reported less pain, stiffness and fatigue, and fewer nights of difficult sleeping. These findings may relate to increased serotonin levels, as increased serotonin levels have been noted in other conditions following massage therapy (Ironson et al 1996). Low serotonin levels may contribute to the non-restorative sleep, mood alteration and increased pain sensitivity noted in fibromyalgia patients (Russell 1989). The purpose of this study was to determine whether massage therapy increased restorative sleep, decreased substance P levels, and reduced pain.

Method

Participants

Twenty adult patients were recruited from a local university and were randomly assigned to a massage therapy or relaxation therapy group. They averaged 9 years in treatment. The two groups did not differ on age, socio-economic status or ethnicity.

Procedure

Massage therapy   Participants received a massage twice a week for 5 weeks by a volunteer professional massage therapist. The massage consisted of moderate-pressure stroking of the head, neck, shoulders, back, arms, hands, legs and feet for 30 minutes. The massage began with lengthening and stretching of the neck and spine with the hands positioned under the head and neck followed by stroking the forehead and face. Pressure was applied to the tender points, and the shoulders were gently depressed. The arms and legs were stretched, and the arms were lifted and moved in a circular motion. Finger pressure was applied to the palms of the hands and the soles of the feet with extra pressure given to the tender points. Stroking was then continued from the top to the bottom of the limbs. Medium-pressure squeezing was applied to the upper shoulder and neck area, while light, brisk rubbing movements were performed along the spine. The massage was concluded in each position with gentle rocking and more stroking from head to toe.

Progressive muscle relaxation therapy   A relaxation group was assessed to control for potential placebo effects or improvement related to the increased attention given to the massage therapy group participants. The relaxation therapy group was given instructions on how to conduct progressive muscle relaxation sessions for 30 minutes while lying quietly on the massage table, including tensing and relaxing large muscle groups starting with the head, neck, shoulders, back, arms, hands, legs, and feet. The therapist conducted these sessions twice a week for 5 weeks with the participants.

Assessments (before and after treatment sessions on the first and last days)   The State Anxiety Inventory (STAI) (Spielberger et al 1970) is an anxiety scale consisting of 20 items on how the participant feels at that moment in terms of severity from (1) 'not at all' to (4) 'very much so'. Typical items include 'I feel nervous' and 'I feel calm'. The Profile of Mood States (McNair et al 1971) is a five-point adjective-rating scale on how well an adjective describes the participants' feelings including helpless or gloomy feelings, depression and anxiety.

Assessments of longer–term effects   The Center for Epidemiological Studies Depression Scale (CES-D) (Radloff 1977) is a 20-item questionnaire that measures depressive symptoms over the past week. Characteristic items include 'I felt depressed', 'I had crying spells', and 'I did not feel like eating, my appetite was poor'. A motion recorder, a Timex watch with the time mechanism removed so that each limb movement advanced the time hand of the watch, was worn to record activity during sleep. The watch's reading was recorded at bedtime and at rise time. The physician's assessment included tender points and pain as assessed by a dolorimeter. The point pressure threshold was measured by exerting increasing force over the 18 tender point sites. Saliva samples collected before the first and last sessions were assayed for substance P. Saliva was obtained from a cotton dental swab coated with lemonade crystals by placing it in the participant's mouth until it was saturated with saliva. The saliva was then transferred into a microcentrifuge tube with a syringe and frozen for later analysis at Children's Hospital of Philadelphia.

Results

As can be seen in Table 8.4, across the course of the study, the massage therapy group as compared with the relaxation group experienced decreased depression, improved sleep (a greater number of hours sleeping and fewer sleep movements), decreased symptoms including pain, a decrease in the number of tender points, and a reduced substance P level (Fig. 8.8).

Discussion

The decrease in anxiety and depressed mood after massage therapy, less depression and pain were consistent with our previous findings with fibromyalgia (Sunshine et al 1996). Using a motion recorder confirmed the previous findings of less difficulty sleeping (Sunshine et al 1996). Less difficulty sleeping and less sleep activity may have contributed to the decrease in substance P (Sunshine et al 1996).

STUDY 4: CARPAL TUNNEL SYNDROME SYMPTOMS ARE LESSENED FOLLOWING MASSAGE THERAPY

The incidence of carpal tunnel syndrome has significantly increased since the advent of the computer (Martin 2000) and continues to contribute to unpleasant symptoms, loss of worker productivity and worker's compensation costs. Carpal tunnel syndrome is defined as pain and paresthesias (tingling, burning, and numbness) in the hand in the area of the median nerve by bounded fibers

Table 8.4 Means for long-term effects of massage therapy

Measure	First day massage	Last day massage	First day massage	Last day massage
Depression	18.0[a]	12.3[b]	17.7[a]	17.1[a]
Sleep hours	5.8[a]	6.4[b]	5.6[a]	6.2[a]
Sleep movements	101.3[a]	83.3[b]	86.1[b]	74.6[b]
Pain	6.0[a]	3.7[b]	7.7[a]	6.3[a]
Physical assessment of pain	4.5[a]	3.3[b]	5.3[a]	4.8[a]
Substance P	84.1[a]	69.2[b]	71.9[b]	111.1[c]

[a,b,c]Different superscripts denote significant differences.

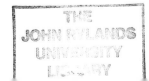

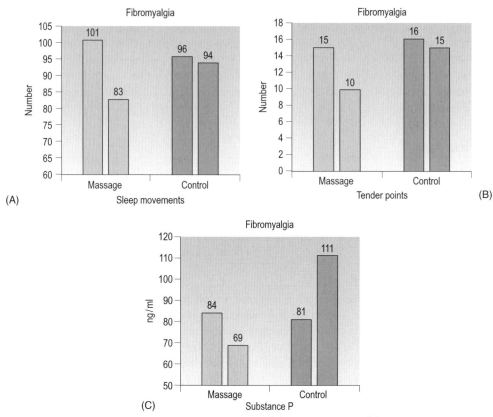

(A)

(B)

(C)

Figure 8.8 Massage therapy group experienced (A) improved sleep, (B) a decrease in the number of tender points, and (C) reduced substance P levels, as compared to the control group.

of the carpal ligament (Akelman & Weiss 1995, Kulick 1996), and local metabolic dysfunction of the median nerve causes a nerve conduction delay (Akelman & Weiss 1995). The diagnosis typically is based on clinical symptoms and signs, including Tinel and Phalen signs (D'Arcy & McGee 2000). Interventions include splints, non-steroidal anti-inflammatory agents, and steroid injections.

The carpal tunnel release procedure, which is among the top 10 operating room procedures, accounting for $1 billion in direct medical costs, has been generally successful in approximately 75% of cases (Blanc et al 1996). However, complications have accompanied this procedure including failure to completely divide the transverse carpal ligament, injury to the median nerve, scarring, loss of motion, and a recurrence rate in about 9–19% of cases (Lindau & Karlsson 1999). Exercise and yoga (Seradge et al 2000) programs have resulted in as much as a 45% reduction in carpal tunnel syndrome symptoms. Low-level laser acupuncture and transcutaneous electrical nerve stimulation have also reduced carpal tunnel syndrome pain (Braco & Naeser 1999).

Self-massage appears to be a technique that people naturally use (rubbing with pressure) to reduce pain. Massage therapy has reduced pain in other syndromes such as fibromyalgia (Sunshine et al 1996) and low back pain (Hernandez-Reif et al 2001), and massage therapy increases serotonin levels, known to reduce pain. The current study examined massage therapy effects on pain, median nerve conduction, and accompanying anxiety and depression related to carpal tunnel syndrome (Field et al 2004).

Method

Participants

Sixteen adults were recruited at a local university via advertising for people already diagnosed as having carpal tunnel syndrome whose work involved extensive time at the computer. The number of years since diagnosis averaged 6.7, and 23% had experienced surgery. The diagnosis of carpal tunnel syndrome was made again based upon the participant's complaints and physical findings (positive Phalen's tests and Tinel sign). The participants were then randomly assigned to standard treatment control and massage therapy groups. The groups did not differ on the above variables.

Procedure

The massage therapy group participants received a massage on the affected arm by a therapist once a week for a 4-week period and were also taught self-massage that was to be done daily at home prior to bedtime. The participants were called on a weekly basis to check on their scheduling daily sessions. The 15-minute massage consisted of moderate-pressure stroking concentrated on the fingertip-to-elbow area. The massage began with stroking the wrist up to the elbow and back down on both sides of the forearm. Next, a wringing motion (much like milking a cow) was applied to the same area. This was followed by stroking, using the thumb and forefinger, in a circular or back-and-forth motion covering the entire forearm and hand. Finally, the skin was rolled using the thumb and forefinger across the hand and up both sides of the forearm.

The massage group participants were asked to complete a massage and pain log for the month. The participants were asked to use the log to report the time they started and finished the self-massage as well as their level of pain at that time using a scale from 0 to 10 with 0 being no pain and 10 being the most intense pain.

The standard treatment control group received the same assessments as the massage group but did not receive massage therapy during the study. They were taught the self-massage routine after the end of the study.

Physicians' assessments   The collaborating physicians assessed the participants at the beginning and end of the study on the following:

- Carpal tunnel symptoms including loss of strength, tingling, numbness, burning or pain to the affected area.
- The Tinel sign, elicited by lightly tapping the carpal ligament over the median nerve along the wrist. For a positive sign, the person feels a pain or tingling sensation along the thumb or first two fingers.
- The Phalen test, requiring the participants to flex their wrists firmly with both palms touching at a 90° angle for 60 seconds. The same process is done inversely with the back of the hands touching. The test is positive if numbness or tingling sensations are experienced along the path of the median nerve across the wrist and hand.
- Nerve conduction test. Nerve conduction velocity of the median nerve was measured using a device that can perform electromyography as well as nerve conduction testing. Stimulation of the median nerve is proximal to distal for the motor response and distal to proximal for the sensory studies. Stimulation of the median sensory nerves was accomplished using ring electrodes placed on the index finger with the recording electrode placed at a fixed distance of 12–14 cm on the flexor surface of the wrist. A ground electrode was placed on the dorsum of the hand being evaluated. Peak sensory latencies were obtained. Latencies greater than 3.6 ms were considered to be prolonged (abnormal) and suggest nerve compression at the carpal tunnel when commensurate with appropriate signs and symptoms. Motor conductions were performed with the stimulating electrodes placed at the flexor surface of the wrist (region over the median nerve) with the active recording electrode over the belly of the abductor policis brevis muscle and the indifferent electrode just distal to the first metacarpophalengeal joint. The compound action potential was recorded after stimulation at the wrist 7–10 cm from the active electrode and at the antecubital fossa 15–20 cm from the distal stimulating electrode. The latencies obtained were subtracted and divided into the distance between the proximal and distal latencies to provide a velocity. A velocity below 48.0 m/s was considered to be slow (abnormal) and suggests neuropraxia (mildest form of nerve block associated with reversible injury).

Pre-/post-session assessments   The participants completed the following assessments before and after the treatment sessions on the first and last days of the 1-month study:

- Perceived Grip Strength scale is a 10-point scale, ranging from weakest (score of 0) to strongest (score of 10) grip, where the participants determine their perceived grip strength after clenching both fists for 5 seconds.
- VITAS (VITAS Healthcare Corporation, FL, USA) is a pre-/post-session pain assessment using a visual analog scale (VAS) ranging from 0 (no pain) to 10 (worst possible pain), anchored with five faces.
- The State Anxiety Inventory (STAI) (Spielberger et al 1970) consists of 20 items on how the participant feels at that moment in terms of severity from 1 = 'not at all' to 4 = 'very much so'. Typical items include 'I feel nervous' and 'I feel calm'.

- The Profile of Mood States (POMS; McNair et al 1971) is a five-point Likert rating scale on how well an adjective describes the participant's feelings including helpless or gloomy feelings, depression and anxiety.

Results

The massage therapy group showed fewer carpal tunnel symptoms and a shorter median peak latency by the end of the treatment period (see Table 8.5). Improvement was also noted for the massage therapy group on the Phalen test and nerve conduction velocity measures.

Functional activity also improved including reduced pain and increased grip strength in the massage therapy group, both immediately after the first and last massage therapy sessions and by the end of the study (see Table 8.6). Finally, the massage therapy group reported lower anxiety and depressed

Table 8.5   Means for physicians' assessments (control group in parentheses)

Measure	First day	Last day
Carpal tunnel symptoms	3.00	2.22[a]
	(3.00)	(3.00)
Tinel's sign	3.11	3.11
	(3.33)	(3.33)
Phalen test	2.67	3.00[a]
	(2.33)	(2.50)
Nerve conduction velocity	46.79	53.57[a]
	(46.49)	(49.24)
Median peak latency	3.59	3.40[a]
	(3.50)	(3.48)

[a] $p < 0.05$.

Table 8.6   Means for pre-/post-session measures (control group in parentheses)

Measures	First day		Last day	
	Pre-	Post-	Pre-	Post-
Pain (VITAS)	4.11	2.22[a]	2.59[b]	0.96[c]
	(6.17)	(6.16)	(4.83)	(5.33)
Grip strength	6.61	8.80[2]	7.80[b]	8.98[d]
	(5.58)	(5.00)	(6.25)	(6.08)
Anxiety (STAI)	35.11	25.62[a]	31.89[b]	25.69[a]
	(31.00)	(26.17)	(32.50)	(31.33)
Depression (POMS)	5.44	1.89[d]	3.95[b]	2.22[d]
	(4.17)	(2.50)	(3.50)	(3.50)

Superscripts in columns 2 and 4 indicate pre-/post-differences and in column 3 indicate first day–last day differences. [a] $p < 0.005$, [b] $p < 0.05$, [c] $p < 0.001$, [d] $p < 0.01$.

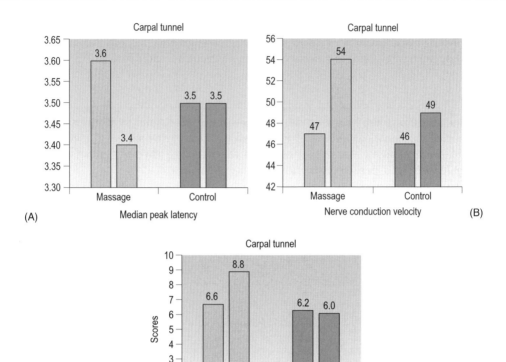

Figure 8.9 The massage therapy group showed (A) a shorter median peak latency, (B) improvement on nerve conduction velocity measures, and (C) increased grip strength.

mood levels both immediately after the first and last sessions and by the end of the study (Table 8.6).

Discussion

Several underlying mechanisms have been hypothesized for pain reduction following massage therapy, including the gate theory (Tennent & Goddard 1997), which suggests that larger, more myelinated fibers such as pressure fibers transmit the pressure message more rapidly to the brain than the smaller less myelinated pain fibers, thus 'closing the gate' to the pain message. Other potential mechanisms are the release of pain-relieving neurotransmitters such as serotonin and oxytocin. Serotonin has been noted to increase following massage therapy in several pain syndromes (Field 1998), and oxytocin has been noted to increase following massage and acupuncture in the rat model (Uvnas-Moberg 1994). The reduction in carpal tunnel symptoms and in median peak latency probably also derive from the stimulation of pressure receptors.

The increase in grip strength could be related to massage increasing muscle strength or simply grip strength increasing as pain is decreased. Finally, decreases in self-reported anxiety and depression invariably occur following massage therapy associated decreases in pain (Field 1998), so these effects were not surprising.

Future research is needed for replication of these effects with a better control group (e.g. a group that receives some form of physical contact) and for exploring underlying mechanisms. Other electrophysiological tests of more chronic symptoms, for example, sleep disturbances and neurotransmitter/neurohormone assays may help inform the process of pain reduction following massage therapy.

References

Akelman E, Weiss AP 1995 Carpal tunnel syndrome: etiology and endoscopic treatment. The Orthopedic Clinics of North America 26:769–778.

Beckelew S, Conway R, Parker J, et al 1998 Biofeedback/relaxation training and exercise interventions for fibromyalgia: a prospective trial. Arthritis Care and Resarch 11:196–209.

Bergstrom KA, Jolkkonen J, Kuikka JT, et al 1998 Fentanyl decreases beta-CIT binding to the dopamine transporter. Synapse 29:413–415.

Berman B, Swyers J, Ezzo J 2000 The evidence for acupuncture as a treatment for rheumatological conditions. Rheumatic Diseases Clinics of North America 26:103–115.

Blanc PD, Faucett J, Kennedy J et al 1996 Self-reported carpal tunnel syndrome: predictors of work disability from the National Health Interview Survey Occupational Health Supplement. American Journal of Industrial Medicine 30:362–368.

Braco K, Naeser MA 1999 Carpal tunnel syndrome: clinical outcome after low-level laser acupuncture, microamps transcutaneous electrical nerve stimulation, and other alternative therapies—an open protocol study. Journal of Alternative and Complementary Medicine 5:5–26.

Courtney T, Webster B 1999 Disabling occupational morbidity in the United States. An alternative way of seeing the Bureau of Labor Statistics' data. Journal of Occupational and Environmental Medicine 41:60–69.

D'Arcy CA, McGee S 2000 Does this patient have carpal tunnel syndrome? Journal of the American Medical Association 283:3110–3117.

Ernst E 1999 Massage therapy for low back pain: a systematic review. Journal of Pain and Symptom Management 17(1):65–69.

Field T 1998 Massage therapy effects. American Psychologist 53:1270–1281.

Field T, Grizzle N, Scafidi F, et al 1996 Massage therapy for infants of depressed mothers. Infant Behavior and Development 19:1107–1112.

Field T, Hernandez-Reif M, Quintino O, et al 1997a Elder retired volunteers benefit from giving massage therapy to infants. Journal of Applied Gerontology 17:229–239.

Field T, Sunshine W, Hernandez-Reif M, et al 1997b Massage therapy effects on depression and somatic symptoms in chronic fatigue immunodeficiency syndrome. Journal of Chronic Fatigue Syndrome 3:43–51.

Field T, Hernandez-Reif M, Seligman S, et al 1997c Juvenile rheumatoid arthritis benefits from massage therapy. Journal of Pediatric Psychology 22:607–617.

Field T, Diego M, Cullen C, et al 2002 Fibromyalgia pain and substance P decrease and sleep improves after massage therapy. Journal of Clinical Rheumatology 8:72–76.

Field T, Delage J, Hernandez-Reif M 2003 Movement and massage therapy reduce fibromyalgia pain. Journal of Bodywork and Movement Therapies 7:49–52.

Field T, Diego M, Cullen C, et al 2004 Carpal tunnel syndrome symptoms are lessened following massage therapy. Journal of Bodywork and Movement Therapies 8:9–14.

Hernandez-Reif M, Field T, Krasnegor J, et al 2000 Lower back pain is reduced and range of motion increased after massage therapy. International Journal of Neuroscience 106:131–145.

Hernandez-Reif M, Field T, Largie B, et al 2001 Children's distress during burn treatment is reduced by massage therapy. Journal of Burn Care & Rehabilitation 22:191–195.

Ironson G, Field T, Scafidi F, et al 1996 Massage therapy is associated with the enhancement of the immune system's cytotoxic capacity. International Journal of Neuroscience 84:205–217.

Jhingran P, Cady RK, Rubino J, et al 1996 Improvments in health-related quality of life with sumatriptan treatment for migraine. Journal of Family Practice 42:36–42.

Juhl J 1998 Fibromyalgia and the serotonin pathway. Alternative Medicine Review 3:367–375.

Kulick RG 1996 Carpal tunnel syndrome. Orthopedic Clinics of North America 27:345–354.

Latarjet J, Choinere M 1995 Pain in burn patients. Burns 21:344–348.

Lindau T, Karlsson MK 1999 Complications and outcome in open carpal tunnel release. Chirurgie de la Main 18:115–121.

McGrath P, Johnson G, Goodman J, et al 1985 CHEOPS: a behavioral scale for rating postoperative pain in children. Advances in Pain Research and Therapy 9:395–402.

McNair DM, Lorr M, Droppleman LF 1971 POMS - Profile of Mood States. Educational and Industrial Testing Service, San Diego, CA.

Martin DS 2000 A rational approach to the management of carpal tunnel syndrome in the workplace. Tennessee Medicine: Journal of the Tennessee Medical Association 93:205–207.

Moldofsky H 1993 A chronobiologic theory of fibromyalgia. Journal of Musculoskeletal Pain 1: 49–59.

Mooney V, Saal JA, Saal JS 1996 Evaluation and treatment of low back pain. Clinical Symposia 48:1–32.

Nicholas MK, Wilson PH, Goyen J 1992 Comparison of cognitive-behavioral group treatment and an alternative non-psychological treatment for chronic low back pain. Pain 48:339–347.

Radloff L 1977 The CES-D scale: a self-report depression scale for research in the general population. Applied Psychological Measurement 1:385–401.

Russell I 1989 Neurohormonal aspects of fibromyalgia syndrome. Rheumatic Diseases Clinics of North America 15:149–168.

Russell I, Michalek J, Vipraio J, et al 1992 Platelet 3H-imipramine uptake receptor density and serum serotonin levels in patients with fibromyalgia/fibrositis symptoms. Journal of Rheumatology 19:104–119.

Russell I, Orr M, Littman B, et al 1994 Elevated cerebrospinal fluid levels of substance P in patients with fibromyalgia syndrome. Arthritis and Rheumatism 37:1593–1601.

Seradge H, Bear C, Bithell D 2000 Preventing carpal tunnel syndrome and cumulative trauma disorder: effect of carpal tunnel decompression excercises: an Oklahoma experience. Journal of Oklahoma State Medical Association 93:150–153.

Snyder-Halpern R, Verran JA 1987 Instrumentation to describe subjective sleep
characteristics in healthy subjects. Research in Nursing & Health 10:155–163.

Solomon GD, Skobieranda FG, Genzen JR 1995 Quality of life assessment among
migraine patients treated with sumatriptan. Headache 35(8):449–454.

Spielberger CD, Gorusch RC, Lushene RE 1970 The State Trait Anxiety Inventory.
Consulting Psychologists Press, Palo Alto, CA.

Sunshine W, Field T, Quintino O, et al 1996 Massage therapy and transcutaneous
electrical stimulation effects on fibromyalgia. Journal of Clinical Rheumatology
2:18–22.

Tennent TD, Goddard NJ 1997 Carpal tunnel decompression: open vs endoscopic. British
Journal of Hospital Medicine 58:551–554.

Uvnas-Moberg K, Widstrom A, Marchini G, et al 1987 Release of GI hormones in mother
and infant by sensory stimulation. Acta Paediatrica Scandinavica 76:851–860.

Verran J, Snyder-Halperin R 1988 Do patients sleep in the hospital? Applied Nursing
Research 1(2):95.

Chapter 9

Enhancing immune function

In several studies, natural killer cells have been noted to increase following massage therapy. It suggests improved immune function, given that natural killer cells are the front line of the immune system, warding off viral cells and cancer cells. In a study on HIV-affected adolescents, natural killer cells were noted to increase following a period of massage. This suggested a better clinical course as a natural killer cells have been noted to substitute for CD4 cells, the cells that are destroyed in HIV. In this study the CD4 cells were also increased, showing a little indication of improved clinical condition for these adolescents. In a similar study on leukemia in children, lymphocytes and another index of improved immune function, were noted to increase following a period of massage therapy. This change indicated improved clinical condition in the children with leukemia. In a study on breast cancer, natural killer cells were again shown to increase, suggesting improved immune function.

STUDY 1: ADOLESCENTS WITH HIV SHOW IMPROVED IMMUNE FUNCTION FOLLOWING MASSAGE THERAPY

HIV is a complex retrovirus that primarily affects the human immune system by attacking CD4 and T cells. Shortly after HIV infection and the abrupt decline in immune function, acute infections disappear leaving the person asymptomatic, sometimes for years, before the onset of opportunistic infections, AIDS and death (CDC 1997). Pharmacological interventions, typically consisting of a combination of antiretroviral drugs, have been expensive, difficult to adhere to and often accompanied by severe side-effects (Abrams 1997).

Although much progress has been made in slowing down the progression of HIV, there is still no available cure or vaccine. This, along with the expense and severe side-effects of antiretroviral drugs has led over half of HIV-infected Americans to try some form of alternative medicine (Abrams 1997). Data from an Office of Alternative Medicine (OAM)-sponsored study reveals that up to 60% of those receiving alternative treatments for HIV receive massage therapy (Reeves et al 1998). A recent research study on the effects of massage therapy on immunodeficiency supports this. In this HIV study, men who were HIV+ showed increased natural killer (NK) cell number and cytotoxicity (activity) following an intensive 1-month-long massage therapy intervention (Ironson et al 1996). Increases in natural killer cells have been shown to provide protection against common AIDS diseases such as tumors and viruses (Whiteside & Herberman 1989).

Similar increases in NK cells were found in another study involving 20 women with Stage I or II breast cancer who had undergone a mastectomy and were subsequently given massage therapy (Hernandez-Reif et al 2005). Unfortunately the study on massage therapy in HIV men did not result in altered disease markers, CD4 number and CD4/CD8 ratio, probably because treatment only lasted for 1 month.

The present study (Diego et al 2001) determined whether the disease markers, CD4 number and CD4/CD8 ratio would be altered by massage therapy in a sample where:

- the participants were randomly assigned to either a massage therapy or a relaxation therapy control group to eliminate the confounding factors associated with within-subjects designs;
- the treatment period was longer, lasting 3 months rather than 5 weeks;
- the treatment sessions were less intensive, consisting of partial body chair massages versus full-body table massages, two rather than five times per week for 20 versus 45 minutes, to assess whether a less intensive treatment regime could alter immune function;
- most of the participants were female and younger (13–19 years).

Method

Participants

Twenty-four HIV-seropositive adolescents (22 females) were recruited from an Adolescent Health Care Service at the medical school of the University of Miami. The adolescents had a mean CD4 number of $466/mm^3$, and they did not differ in their anti-HIV drug regimens and did not undergo any changes in drug regimens during the period of the therapy sessions.

Procedure

The participants were randomly assigned to a massage therapy or a relaxation therapy group. The first day of therapy was scheduled within a week of the subject's regularly scheduled blood draw, and the last day of therapy was scheduled within a week before the subject's next regularly scheduled blood draw (12 weeks later) to eliminate immune assay expenses. In addition, before and after the sessions, on the first and last days of the study, the participants were asked to complete the following assessments: a demographic questionnaire, the Center for Epidemiological Studies on Depression Scale (CES-D), and the State Anxiety Inventory.

Massage therapy The adolescents in the massage therapy group received a 20-minute massage therapy session by professional massage therapists (different therapist each session), while sitting fully clothed in a standard massage chair. The therapist administered a standard chair massage procedure that consisted of long broad strokes with moderate pressure to the:

Back:

1. compression to the back parallel to the spine from the shoulders to the base of the spine;
2. compression to the entire back adding gentle rocking;
3. squeezing of the shoulder and upper arm muscles;
4. finger pressure to shoulder;
5. finger pressure along the length of the spine and back;
6. circular strokes to the hips.

Arms:

1. arms dropped to the side. Arms kneaded from shoulder to lower arm;
2. pressing down on upper and lower arms.

Hands:

1. entire hands massaged and gentle pulling of fingers;
2. the fleshy part of the palm pressed between the thumb and index finger for 15 to 20 seconds;
3. gentle pulling of the arms in both lateral and superior directions.

Neck:

1. kneading the neck;
2. finger pressure along base of skull and along side of neck;
3. scalp massage;
4. pressing down on trapezius, finger pressure and squeezing continuing down the arms.

Relaxation therapy The adolescents in this group were guided through a 20-minute progressive muscle relaxation routine by a research assistant or a massage therapist (different therapist each session) two times per week for 12 weeks, 20 minutes each session. The routine consisted of asking the adolescents to sit on a comfortable sofa. Then the therapist with a calm and soothing voice instructed the adolescent to successively tense and relax muscles in each of the same areas that were massaged in the massage group (back, arms, hands, and neck). Progressive muscle relaxation was successfully used as a control condition in a number of studies that have evaluated the effects of massage therapy (Field et al 1992, Hernandez-Reif et al 2005).

Short-term assessments State Anxiety Inventory (STAI; Spielberger et al 1970) is a 20-item scale that measures the transitory anxiety levels in terms of severity, with 1 = 'not so much' and 4 = 'very much'. Characteristic items include 'I feel tense' and 'I feel relaxed'.

Longer-term assessments Center for Epidemiological Studies Depression Scale (CES-D; Radloff 1977) is a 20-item questionnaire, with possible scores between 0 and 60. The respondents rate the frequency (within the last week) of 20 symptoms. The symptoms include depressed mood, feelings of helplessness and hopelessness, feelings of guilt and worthlessness, loss of energy, and problems with sleep and appetite.

Immune measures were obtained from the medical charts after the adolescents' regularly scheduled clinic blood draw (every 12 weeks). Samples were assayed for the HIV disease progression markers inculding: T-helper cells (CD4 number); T-suppressor cells (CD8+ number); and CD4/CD8 ratio. Natural killer cells were also assayed as they have been shown to protect against common AIDS diseases including tumors and viruses (Whiteside & Herberman 1989).

Results

Data analyses revealed that both groups reported a decrease in anxiety immediately after treatment on both the first and last days. Tests conducted on the depression scale (CES-D) scores revealed that only the massage therapy group reported a decrease in depression (Table 9.1). The analyses revealed an increase in CD4 count in the massage therapy group only (Fig. 9.1A), as well as an increase in CD4/CD8. Natural killer cell number also increased significantly, but only for the massage therapy group (Table 9.2, Fig. 9.1B).

Table 9.1   Mean depression and anxiety scores

	Massage				Control			
	First day		Last day		First day		Last day	
	Pre–	Post–	Pre–	Post–	Pre–	Post–	Pre–	Post–
State anxiety	44[a]	30[b]	39[a]	27[b]	42[a]	35[b]	41[a]	36[b]
Depression	26[a]		15[b]		24[a]		22[a]	

[a,b]Different superscript letters denote differences between means.

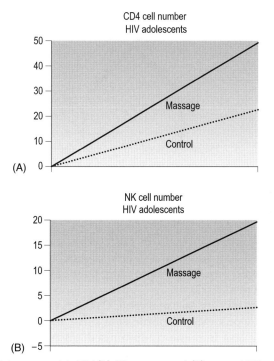

Figure 9.1   In adolescents with HIV (A) CD4 count and (B) natural killer cell number increased in the massage therapy group.

Discussion

HIV infection is commonly accompanied by depression and anxiety, which might result in the production of cortisol, which would further suppress the immune system and NK cells in particular (Lutgendorf et al 1996). Although we did not measure cortisol in this study, the positive massage therapy effects on NK cell number and activity might be explained by reduced stress, anxiety and cortisol following massage therapy (see Fig. 9.2 for a proposed mechanism). Lowered cortisol would result in increased NK cell number and activ-

Table 9.2   Means for immune measures

Measure	Massage (n = 12)		Control (n = 12)	
	Pre–	Post–	Pre–	Post–
Natural killer cell (n)	133[a]	160[b]	137[a]	135[a]
CD4 (n)	467[a]	506[b]	465[a]	479[a]
CD8 (n)	765[a]	755[a]	877[a]	827[a]
CD4/CD8 ratio	0.61[a]	0.67[b]	0.53[a]	0.58[a]

[a,b]Different superscript letters denote differences between means.

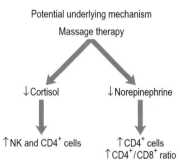

Figure 9.2   Potential underlying mechanism for the effects of massage on natural killer cell number and CD4 count.

ity, signifying an important gain in HIV (Whiteside & Herberman 1989). Others have noted that in advanced HIV cases characterized by low CD4 counts, persons who remain asymptomatic may have greater NK cell functioning (Solomon et al 1993).

The effect on the HIV disease marker (CD4/CD8 ratio) shown in this study but not in our previous study (Ironson et al 1996), might be explained by the adolescents being less immune-compromised. Also the adolescents in this study had high levels of depression. Depression has been linked to immunosuppression through decreased CD4 number and CD4/CD8 ratio (Ravindram et al 1995). Massage therapy then by reducing depression might improve CD4/CD8 ratio and CD4 number in HIV-infected adolescents.

STUDY 2: LEUKEMIA IMMUNE CHANGES FOLLOWING MASSAGE THERAPY

Children with leukemia can achieve long-term cure and survival (Chessells 2000). However, cancer continues to involve anxiety and depressed mood and compromised immune function. Although adults with leukemia have benefited from relaxation therapy (Arakawa 1997), children are noted to be less compliant with relaxation therapy. For that reason massage therapy may be more effective. Massage therapy would also be indicated for children with leukemia because immune function has been notably enhanced following massage therapy in breast cancer (Hernandez-Reif et al 2004).

The present study assessed the effects of massage therapy on anxiety, depressed mood and immune function in children with leukemia (Field et al 2001). The parents were taught the massage so that the therapy could be provided on a daily basis, would be cost-effective and might reduce the parents' depressed mood.

Method

Participants and procedure

Twenty children with leukemia participated in this study. The children who were referred by a pediatric oncologist were randomly assigned to the massage therapy or a wait list control group. The parents were guided through the 15-minute massage by having them practice it on their child under the direction of a massage therapist. The parents were instructed to give the massage before bedtime every day for 30 days. The 15-minute massage consisted of applying moderate pressure on the face, neck, shoulders, back, stomach, legs, feet, arms and hands.

For the first phase, the child was in a supine position, and oil was applied to ensure smooth, continuous stroking movements. The parents stroked the child's body in the following sequence:

Face:

1. stroking along both sides of the face;
2. flats of fingers across the forehead;
3. circular flat stroking over the nose, cheeks, jaw, and chin.

Stomach:

1. hand-over-hand stroking in a paddlewheel fashion, avoiding the ribs and the tip of the rib cage;
2. circular motion with fingers in a clockwise direction starting at the appendix.

Legs:

1. stroking from the hip to foot;
2. squeezing and twisting in a wringing motion from hip to foot;
3. massaging foot and toes;
4. stretching the Achilles tendon;
5. stroking the legs upward to the heart.

Arms:

1. stroking from the shoulders to the hands;
2. same procedure as for the legs.

For the second phase, with the child in a prone position, the back was massaged in the following sequence:

1. downward stroking along the back;
2. hand-over-hand movements from the upper back to the buttocks;
3. hands from side to side across the back, including the sides;
4. circular motion from the head to the buttocks along, but not touching, the spine;
5. simultaneous stroking over the sides of the back from the middle to the sides;
6. rubbing and kneading the shoulder muscles;
7. rubbing the neck;
8. stroking along the length of the back;
9. stroking from the crown to feet.

Wait list control group   The wait list control group parents completed the questionnaires on the first and last days of the study. At the end of the study, the control parents were offered the option of learning the massage.

Pre-/post-session assessments (immediate effects)

These assessments were made before and after the massage therapy and control sessions on the first day of the 30-day study.

Parent assessments

- The State/Trait Anxiety Inventory (STAI; Spielberger et al 1970). The STAI is comprised of 20 items and assesses how the parent feels at that moment in terms of severity (not at all to very much so). Characteristic items include 'I feel nervous' and 'I feel calm'.
- The Profile of Mood States (POMS; McNair et al 1971). The POMS consists of 20 adjectives rating depressed mood at the moment on a five-point scale ranging from 'not at all' to 'extremely' using words such as 'blue', 'sad', and 'miserable'.

Child assessments

- The State Anxiety Inventory for Children (STAIC; Spielberger 1973). The STAIC is an adaptation of the State Anxiety Inventory for assessing anxiety in children consisting of 20 items.
- Profile of Mood States (POMS; McNair et al 1971). This 20-item depression scale (described under parent assessments) was also administered to the children. The scales were read to the child.

First-/last-day assessments (longer-term effects)

Center for Epidemiological Studies Depression Scale (CES–D) (Radloff 1977)   This 20-item scale rates depressive symptoms over the past week on a four-point scale ('rarely or none of the time', 'some or little of the time', 'a lot of the time', and 'most or all of the time').

Complete blood count (CBC)   The complete blood count measures, comprising the white blood count, neutrophil count, and hemoglobin level, were recorded from the child's medical chart on the first and last days of the study.

Results

Data analyses suggested that the massage therapy group parents had lower anxiety and depressed mood levels after the massage therapy sessions on the first day of the study (see Table 9.3). Similarly, the massage therapy group children had lower anxiety and depressed mood levels after the massage therapy sessions on the first day of the study. As can be seen in Table 9.4, the massage therapy group parents' depression decreased from the first to the last day of the study. In addition, the massage group children's white blood count and neutrophil count increased significantly (Fig. 9.3).

Discussion

That the parents' anxiety and depressed mood decreased following their massaging of their child is not surprising inasmuch as similar effects have been reported after elderly volunteers massaged children (Field et al 1998a). Also unsurprising was the decrease in the massaged children's anxiety and depressed mood given similar data for children with other chronic illnesses including asthma (Field et al 1998b) and diabetes (Field et al 1997). The increased white blood count and neutrophil count following massage therapy

Table 9.3   Means for pre-/post-session measures on first day of study for massage therapy group (control group means in parentheses)

	Pre-	Post-
Parent		
Anxiety	33.0^a	27.7^b
	(39.2)	(36.6)
Depressed mood	9.7^a	4.5^b
	(6.9)	(5.9)
Child		
Anxiety	28.0^a	21.7^b
	(29.5)	(27.8)
Depressed mood	8.4^a	3.0^b
	(8.2)	(5.5)

[a,b]Different superscripts denote significant pre-/post-session changes on first day of study for massage therapy group.

Table 9.4   Means for first day/last day measures of massage therapy group (control group means in parentheses)

	First day	Last day
Parent		
Depression	19.0[a]	6.0[b]
	(13.7)	(13.0)
Child		
White blood count	2.5[a]	4.0[b]
	(3.5)	(2.9)
Neutrophils	39.8[a]	52.2[b]
	(40.5)	(35.3)
Hemoglobin	10.5[a]	10.5[a]
	(9.8)	(10.1)

[a,b]Different superscripts denote significant first day/last day changes for massage therapy group.

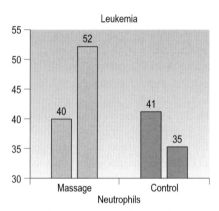

Figure 9.3   In children with leukemia, neutrophil count increased significantly following massage therapy.

suggests the usefulness of this therapy for maintaining optimal immune function over the course of cancer treatment.

STUDY 3: BREAST CANCER PATIENTS HAVE IMPROVED IMMUNE AND NEUROENDOCRINE FUNCTIONS FOLLOWING MASSAGE THERAPY

Psychological stress has been associated with lower NK cell number and lower NK cell activity in women with breast cancer (Levy et al 1987). Reduced NK cell numbers may present a significant problem inasmuch as these cells play an important role in anti-cancer defense (Brittenden et al 1996, Locke et al 1984). Breast cancer patients have reduced NK cell number (Brittenden et al 1996), and stress further decreases NK cell activity (Ben-Eliyahu et al 1999, Brittenden et al 1996). Massage therapy has been shown to increase NK cell number and NK cell activity in men (Ironson et al 1996) and adolescents with HIV (Diego et al 2001). Massage therapy has also been associated with improved mood and increased serotonin (5-HIAA) and dopamine levels, which would increase NK cells (Field 1998).

The specific aim of this study was to assess the effects of 5 weeks of massage therapy on serotonin, dopamine, and NK cell number compared to the control group (Hernandez-Reif et al 2005). The inclusion criteria included: stage I or II breast cancer diagnosis within the past 3 years, and at least 3 months post-surgery, -chemotherapy and/or -radiation therapy, because radiation and chemotherapy affect immune measures.

Method

Participants

The sample comprised 34 women who had been diagnosed with stage I or II breast cancer. The women were randomly assigned to a massage therapy group or a standard treatment control group (n = 16) using a flip of a coin. The groups did not differ on stage of cancer, type of surgery, treatments received, or demographic variables.

Procedure

The 30-minute massage routine consisted of Swedish, Trager and Acupressure techniques. The massage sessions followed a standardized protocol that was similar to the protocol that had been effective in reducing stress hormones and increasing NK cells in our HIV study (Ironson et al 1996).

With the participant covered in a supine position and the therapist standing at the head of the massage table, the following techniques were applied:

Head/neck (2 minutes):

- stretching of the neck;
- lateral stroking of the forehead;
- stroking and stretching of the muscles along the cheeks and jaw;
- depressing the shoulders with the flats of the palms;
- pressing on trigger points at mid-shoulder.

Arms (4 minutes each arm):

- progressive intermittent compressions from the axillary region (armpit) to the chest (six times); intermittent compression of the arm, beginning at the shoulder and increasing 4–6 inches of the arm and returning to shoulder each time before the addition of another section until the entire arm from the shoulder to the wrist has been included;

- broad circular movements with the flats of the hand to the chest from the sternum to the shoulder;
- long strokes (using oil) from the sternum to the shoulder and from the wrist to the shoulder;
- slow range of motion of the arm including full arm flexion (overhead), abduction, horizontal adduction and abduction and rotation of the humerus.

Standing at the foot of the massage table, the therapist delivered the following:

Legs/feet (4 minutes each leg):

- pulling (or traction) of both legs and each leg separately;
- massage of the feet, including squeezing of the heel;
- long gliding strokes up the leg from ankle to knee;
- kneading of the thigh muscles; long strokes from the hip to the foot.

With the participant in a prone position with a towel or small flat cushion under the breast area for comfort, the following steps were performed:

Legs (3 minutes each leg):

- stretching of the Achilles tendon;
- stroking and kneading of the calf muscles;
- long gliding strokes from the heel to the hip;
- rounding strokes to the hip area;
- long strokes from the hip to the feet.

Back (5 minutes):

- using both hands, slow pressing of the muscles of the lower back (10 times);
- long gliding stroking from the lower back to the shoulders and out to the arms;
- squeezing of the trapezius muscles;
- using the outer edge of each hand to perform short strokes along either side of the spine from the neck to the lower back;
- squeezing of the neck muscles;
- long gliding strokes from the shoulders down to the lower back, to the legs and to the feet

Assessments

Anxiety and mood scales were chosen to assess treatment effects: State Trait Anxiety Inventory (STAI) and Profile Mood of States (POMS). On the first and last days of the 5-week session, subjects were asked to complete the SCL-90-R. The SCL-90-R measures depression and anxiety (e.g. 'crying easily', 'loss of sexual interest or pleasure', 'heart pounding or racing', 'feeling tense or keyed-up'). On the morning of the first and the last day of the 5-week study, the women were asked to refrain from eating or drinking and to provide a urine sample. This sample was sent to Duke University for assaying dopamine (activating neurotransmitter) and urinary 5-HIAA (a metabolite of serotonin with lower levels suggestive of depression). The women had their blood drawn to be assayed for NK cell numbers and lymphocytes, which play a role in augmenting the cytotoxicity of NK cells.

Results

The analyses revealed for the massage group (1) reduced anxiety after the first and the last session; (2) reduced depression after the first and last session; and (3) reduced anger (see Table 9.5). The massage therapy group also showed an increase in dopamine and serotonin levels as well as an increase for the massage therapy group in NK cell numbers (Fig. 9.4) and lymphocytes (see Table 9.6).

Table 9.5   Means for anxiety, depression and anger before and after first day and last day sessions

	Massage group				Control group			
	First day		Last day		First day		Last day	
Variables	Pre–	Post–	Pre–	Post–	Pre–	Post–	Pre–	Post–
Immediate effects								
Anxiety	37^a	27^b	35^a	25^b	32^a	30^a	35^a	32^a
Mood								
Depression	12^a	3^b	7^b	3^b	4^b	3^b	6^b	5^b
Anger	10^a	2^b	3^b	2^b	5^b	5^b	3^b	4^b

[a,b]Different letter superscripts indicate differences between pre- and post-session means.

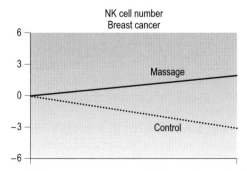

Figure 9.4   In women with breast cancer, natural killer cell number increased following massage therapy.

Table 9.6   Means for longer term measures (first to last day)

	Massage group		Control group	
	First day	Last day	First day	Last day
Depression	13[a]	7[b]	9[a]	11[a]
Anxiety	4[a]	3[a]	4[a]	4[a]
Dopamine	258[a]	325[b]	224[a]	281[a]
Serotonin	2114[a]	3391[b]	3395[b]	3456[b]
NK cell numbers	235[a]	263[b]	254[a]	236[a]
Lymphocytes	29[a]	32[b]	30[a]	30[a]

[a,b]Different letter superscripts indicate differences between first and last day means.

Discussion

The increase in NK cell number supports a previous HIV men's massage therapy study (Ironson et al 1996) and a recent HIV adolescent massage therapy study (Diego et al 2001). Although the effects of massage on immune responses are encouraging, the increases in NK cell activity reported in the HIV men (Ironson et al 1996) and HIV adolescents (Diego et al 2001) studies were not replicated in the current breast cancer group. Perhaps for breast cancer more frequent massages or massage of longer duration would be necessary to achieve a change in NK cell activity.

An improvement in mood is often associated with a change in biochemical levels, and, as expected, the breast cancer patients who received massage therapy showed an increase in dopamine and serotonin levels from the first to the last day of the study. These increases complement the massage group's self-reports of improved mood and decreased depression, as both serotonin and dopamine have been noted to increase in depressed individuals following massage therapy (see Field 1998).

STUDY 4: NATURAL KILLER CELLS AND LYMPHOCYTES ARE INCREASED IN WOMEN WITH BREAST CANCER FOLLOWING MASSAGE THERAPY

One in seven women in the US are likely to develop breast cancer (Weir et al 2003). Women with breast cancer have lower numbers of NK cells (Luecken & Compas 2002, Vgenopoulou et al 2003). Inasmuch as NK cells destroy tumor cells (Brittenden et al 1996), interventions that increase NK cells would benefit women with breast cancer.

Massage therapy has been noted to increase NK cell numbers. In a recent pilot study by our group, women with early stage breast cancer who received massage therapy three times a week for 5 weeks reported reduced anxiety, depression and anger, increased urinary dopamine, serotonin and increased NK cells and lymphocytes (Hernandez-Reif et al 2004).

For the present study, we added women to the massage group of the pilot study and compared the massage group to a relaxation therapy group in order to determine whether the positive effects of our pilot study were due to simple relaxation effects or whether massage itself (i.e. the moderate pressure stimulation of the skin) increased NK cells and lymphocytes (Hernandez-Reif et al 2005). A step effect was predicted, with massage therapy resulting in a greater increase in NK cells than relaxation therapy, which, in turn, was expected to lead to a greater increase than standard treatment alone.

Method

Participants

Fifty-eight women (mean age = 53 years) diagnosed within the past 3 years with early stage (I–III) breast cancer were recruited. The women were assigned to a massage group (n = 22), relaxation group (n = 20) or standard treatment control group (n = 16).

Procedure

Following human subjects review board approval, participants were recruited. Because surgery and radiation therapy have been shown to affect immune measures, participants were not entered into the study until they were at least 3 months post-surgery and/or had completed their last radiation and/or chemotherapy session. At the beginning and at the end of the 5-week study period, participants provided a urine sample, had their blood drawn and completed self-report measures. During the 5-week study period, the women assigned to the massage therapy group received three 30-minute massages each week, and those assigned to progressive muscle relaxation listened to an audiotape describing the step-by-step relaxation procedure, which they practiced at home on the same schedule as the massage therapy group (30-minute sessions, three times a week for 5 weeks).

Therapies

Using unscented massage oil and with the participant in a supine position, the therapist massaged the following areas for 15 minutes:

- Neck/face: lengthening the neck (traction), stroking forehead, circular stroking and stretching jaw area.
- Shoulder: pressing down on the shoulders with the palms of the hands and pressing mid-shoulder trigger points.
- Arms: slow, progressive compressions from the armpit to the chest; compressions along the arm starting at the shoulder and compressing 4–6 inches at a time to the wrist and returning to shoulder again; circular movements with the flat of the hand to the chest from the sternum to the armpit;

and stroking from the sternum to the armpit and from the wrist to the shoulder; range of motion to each arm.

- Torso: placing one hand on the diaphragm, holding and gently rocking.
- Legs/feet: holding both legs together at the heels and then pulling them (traction), as well as pulling the legs together to the right and to the left; massaging the bottom and top of the feet and squeezing the heel; stroking the lower leg from the ankle to the knee; stroking and kneading of the anterior thigh region; stroking from the hip to the foot.

Asking the participant to move into the prone position with a soft pillow under the breast area for comfort, the therapist continued massaging the following areas for 15 minutes:

Legs: flexion and extension of the foot; stroking and kneading the calf muscles; shaking the leg with the knee flexed; stroking from the heel to up and over the buttock; round stroking to the buttock area; stroking from the buttock to the feet.

Back: with the hands positioned on either side of the spine, stretching the back muscles by pressing outward to the sides (10 times) and stroking from the base of the spine to the shoulders and out over the arms; squeezing neck and shoulder areas, using the edge of the hand rubbing alongside the spine from the top to the bottom of the back; squeezing and stretching the neck muscles; pressing on the hip area; stroking from the shoulders down the entire back and legs to the feet.

Progressive Muscle Relaxation (adapted from Bernstein & Borkovec 1973)

The participants assigned to this group practiced progressive muscle relaxation for 15 sessions (three sessions per week for 5 weeks) by following the instructions on a 30-minute audiotape. While taking a deep breath, the participant was asked to tighten the muscles of a particular area for 10 seconds. Then, while letting her breath out, she was asked to relax the muscles and concentrate on how warm the muscles felt when they were relaxed. The relaxation started with the feet and progressed to the calves, thighs, abdomen, hands, arms, back and face in that order.

The Symptom Checklist 90 Revised (SCL-90-R) Depression Subscale (Derogatis 1983)

This is comprised of 15 problems causing distress during the past 7 days (including today) on a Likert scale of 0 (not at all) to 4 (extremely). Characteristic depression problems include 'feeling lonely', 'worrying too much about things', 'feeling no interest in things', 'feelings of worthlessness'.

Neuroendocrine, neurotransmitter and immune function measures

Neuroendocrine and neurotransmitter levels were assayed from urine, and immune assays were carried out on blood samples collected at the beginning and end of the 5-week study. The participants provided fasting blood and urine samples, and to control for diurnal variations, these were collected between 9.00am and 11.00am on the first and last day of the 5-week study period.

Urine assays The urine samples were logged, frozen and sent to Duke University School of Medicine for assaying dopamine and serotonin.

Immune assays These included NK cell number and lymphocytes.

Results

On the SCL-90-R depression score, the massage group had a greater change score on depressive symptoms than the control group. Data analyses revealed increased dopamine and serotonin (5-HIAA) levels for the massage group from the first to the last day (see Table 9.7). The analyses also revealed significant increase in NK cells and lymphocytes for the massage group (see Table 9.8).

Discussion

Only the massage therapy group showed an increase in dopamine and serotonin from the first to the last day of the study. These findings are consistent with other massage studies reporting increased dopamine and increased serotonin levels following massage therapy. The dopamine and serotonin increases may explain the massage group's enduring improved mood in that dopamine and serotonin are activating neurotransmitters.

The pivotal findings in this study were the increases in NK cells and lymphocytes for the women with breast cancer who received massage therapy.

Table 9.7 Mean change score/percent increase or decrease for the urinary measures for the massage therapy, relaxation and control groups

Measures	Massage therapy	Relaxation	Control group
Dopamine (ng/ml)	123/59%[a] ↑	13/14% ↑	57/25% ↑
Serotonin (ng/ml)	837/36%[a] ↑	903/23% ↑	61/2% ↑

[a]Increases are significant.

Table 9.8 Mean change score/percent increase or decrease for the immune measures for the massage therapy, relaxation and control groups

Measures	Massage therapy	Relaxation	Control group
NK cell number	28/12%[a] ↑	22/7% ↑	−18/7% ↓
Lymphocytes	3/9%[a] ↑	0.7/2% ↑	0/0%

[a]Increases are significant.

Their clinical condition would be expected to improve inasmuch as NK cells are noted to destroy tumor cells (Brittenden et al 1996). Stimulation of pressure receptors via massage therapy might be the underlying mechanism for the increased NK cells and lymphocytes. Stimulation of pressure receptors, such as in friction and stroking from massage, may decrease sympathetic and increase parasympathetic activity, leading to enhanced immune function (Diego et al 2004).

References

Abrams D 1997 Dealing with alternative therapies for HIV. In: Sande M, Volberding P (eds) The medical management of AIDS. WB Saunders Co, Philadelphia, PA, pp. 143–158.

Arakawa S 1997 Relaxation to reduce nausea, vomiting, and anxiety induced by chemotherapy in Japanese patients. Cancer 20:342–349.

Ben-Eliyahu S, Page G, Yirmina R, et al 1999 Evidence that stress and surgical interventions promote tumor development by suppressing natural killer cell activity. International Journal of Cancer 80:880–888.

Bernstein B, Borkovec T 1973 Progressive muscle relaxation training: a manual for the helping professions. Research Press, Champaign, IL.

Brittenden J, Heys S, Ross J, et al 1996 Natural killer cells and cancer. Cancer 77:1226–1243.

CDC 1997 HIV/AIDS. Surveillance Report 9(1):1–37.

Chessells J 2000 Recent advances in management of acute leukemia. Archives of the Diseases of Childhood 82:438–442.

Derogatis L 1983 Symptom checklist-90-revised. Administration, scoring, and procedural manual II. Clinical Psychometric Research, New York.

Diego M, Field T, Hernandez-Reif M, et al 2001. HIV adolescents show improved immune function following massage therapy. International Journal of Neuroscience 106:35–45.

Diego M, Field T, Sanders C, et al 2004 Massage therapy of moderate and light pressure and vibrator effects on EEG and heart rate. International Journal of Neuroscience 114:31–44.

Field T 1998 Massage therapy effects. American Psychologist 53:1270–1281.

Field T, Morrow C, Valdeon C, et al 1992 Massage reduces anxiety in child and adolescent psychiatric patients. Journal of the American Academy of Child and Adolescent Psychiatry 31:124–131.

Field T, Hernandez-Reif M, LaGreca A, et al 1997 Massage therapy lowers blood glucose levels in children with diabetes mellitus. Diabetes Spectrum 10:237–239.

Field T, Hernandez-Reif M, Quintino O, et al 1998a Elder retired volunteers benefit from giving massage therapy to infants. Journal of Applied Gerontology 17:229–239.

Field T, Henteleff T, Hernandez-Reif M, et al 1998b Children with asthma have improved pulmonary function after massage therapy. Journal of Pediatrics 132:854–858.

Field T, Cullen C, Diego M, et al 2001 Leukemia immune changes following massage therapy. Journal of Bodywork and Movement Therapies 5:271–274.

Hernandez-Reif M, Ironson G, Field T, et al 2004 Breast cancer patients have improved immune and neuroendocrine functions following massage therapy. Journal of Psychosomatic Research 57:45–52.

Hernandez-Reif M, Field T, Ironson G, et al 2005 Natural killer cells and lymphocytes are increased in women with breast cancer following massage therapy. International Journal of Neuroscience 115(4):495–510.

Ironson G, Field T, Scafidi F, et al 1996 Massage therapy is associated with enhancement of the immune systems cytotoxic capacity. International Journal of Neuroscience 84:205–217.

Levy S, Herberman R, Lippman M, et al 1987 Correlation of stress factors with sustained depression of natural killer cell activity and predicted prognosis in patients with breast cancer. Journal of Clinical Oncology 5:348–353.

Locke S, Kraus L, Leserman J, et al 1984 Life change stress, psychiatric symptoms and natural killer cell activity. Psychosomatic Medicine 46:441–453.

Luecken L, Compas B 2002 Stress, coping and immune function in breast cancer. Annals of Behavioral Medicine 24:336–344.

Lutgendorf S, Antoni M, Shneiderman N, et al 1994 Psychosocial counseling to improve quality of life in HIV infection. Patient Education and Counseling 24:217–235.

McNair D, Lorr M, Droppleman L 1971 Profile of Mood States. Education and Industrial Testing Service, San Diego.

Radloff L 1977 The CES-D scale: a self-report depression scale for research in the general population. Applied Psychological Measurement 1:385–401.

Ravindran A, Griffiths L, Merali Z, et al 1995 Lymphocyte subsets associated with major depression and dysthymia: modification by antidepressant treatment. Psychosomatic Medicine 57:555–563.

Reeves C, Calabrese C, Standish L, et al 1998 Screening alternative therapies for HIV. AIDS Patient Care and STDs 12:87–89.

Solomon G, Benton D, Harker J, et al 1993 Prolonged asymptomatic states in HIV-seropositive persons with CD4 T-cells/mm^3: preliminary psychoimmunologic findings. Journal of Acquired Immunodeficiency Syndromes 6:1173.

Spielberger C 1973 The State-Trait Anxiety Inventory for Children. Consulting Psychological Press, Palo Alto, CA.

Spielberger C, Gorsuch R, Lushen R 1970 The State Anxiety Inventory. Consulting Psychologists Press, Palo Alto, CA.

Vgenopoulou S, Lazaris AC, Markopoulos C, et al 2003 Immunohistochemical evaluation of immune response in invasive ductal breast cancer of not-otherwise-specified type. Breast 12(3):17–28.

Weir HK, Thun MJ, Hankey BF, et al 2003 Annual report to the nation on the status of cancer, 1975–2000, featuring the uses of surveillance data for cancer prevention and control. Journal of the National Cancer Institute 95(17):1276–1299.

Whiteside T, Herberman R 1989 The role of natural killer cells in human disease. Clinical Immunology and Immunopathology 52:1–23.

Appendix 2

Massage therapy abstracts

AGGRESSION

Diego MA, Field T, Hernandez-Reif M, et al (2002). Aggressive adolescents benefit from massage therapy. *Adolescence* **37:597–607**

Method: 17 aggressive adolescents were randomly assigned to a massage therapy group or a relaxation therapy group to receive 20-minute therapy sessions, twice a week for 5 weeks.

Results: The massaged adolescents had lower anxiety after the first and last sessions. By the end of the study, they also reported feeling less hostile and they were perceived by their parents as being less aggressive. Significant differences were not found for the adolescents who were assigned to the relaxation group.

ALZHEIMER'S DISEASE

Rowe M, Alfred D (1999). The effectiveness of slow-stroke massage in diffusing agitated behaviors in individuals with Alzheimer's disease. *Journal of Gerontology and Nursing* **25:22–34**

Method: Agitated behaviors of individuals with Alzheimer's disease (AD), often endured or treated unsuccessfully with chemical or physical restraints, markedly increase the stress levels of family caregivers. The Theoretical Model for Aggression in the Cognitively Impaired guided the examination of caregiver-provided slow-stroke massage on the diffusion of actual and potential agitation for community-dwelling individuals with AD. Characteristics and frequency of agitation were quantified by two highly correlated instruments, the Agitated Behavior Rating Scale Scoring Guide, and the Brief Behavior Symptom Rating Scale.

Results: Expressions of agitation of patients with AD increased in a linear pattern from dawn to dusk. Verbal displays of agitation, the most frequently cited form of agitation in community-dwelling individuals with AD, were not diffused by slow-stroke massage. However, more physical expressions of agitation such as pacing, wandering, and resisting were decreased when slow-stroke massage was applied.

ANOREXIA

Hart S, Field T, Hernandez-Reif M, et al (2001). Anorexia nervosa symptoms are reduced by massage therapy. *Eating Disorders* 9:289–299

Method: Women diagnosed with anorexia nervosa were given a massage twice per week for 5 weeks or standard treatment.

Results: The massaged women reported lower stress and anxiety levels and showed lower cortisol levels immediately following the massage. Over the 5-week treatment period, they also reported decreased body dissatisfaction on the Eating Disorder Inventory and showed increased dopamine and norepinephrine levels. These findings support a previous study on the benefits of massage therapy for eating disorders.

ANXIETY

Field T, Morrow C, Valdeon C, et al (1992). Massage reduces anxiety in child and adolescent psychiatric patients. *Journal of the American Academy of Child and Adolescent Psychiatry* 31:125–131

Method: A 30-minute back massage was given daily for a 5-day period to 52 hospitalized depressed and adjustment disorder children and adolescents.

Results: Compared with a control group who viewed relaxing videotapes, the massage subjects were less depressed and anxious and had lower saliva cortisol levels after the massage. In addition, nurses rated the subjects as being less anxious and more cooperative on the last day of the study, and nighttime sleep increased over this period. Finally, urinary cortisol and norepinephrine levels decreased, but only for the depressed subjects.

McKechnie AA, Wilson F, Watson N, et al (1983). Anxiety states: a preliminary report on the value of connective tissue massage. *Journal of Psychosomatic Research* 27:125–129

Method: Five patients who presented with symptoms of tension and anxiety were subsequently referred to a physiotherapist and treated with connective tissue massage. Psychophysiological recordings of heart rate, frontalis EMG, skin resistance and forearm extensor EMG were taken before and after treatment.

Results: All patients showed a significant response to treatment in one or more of the psychophysiological parameters. Results are discussed in relation to the hypothesis that each individual has a unique stress response pattern.

Shulman KR, Jones GE (1996). The effectiveness of massage therapy intervention on reducing anxiety in the work place. *Journal of Applied Behavioral Science* **32:160–173**

Method: An on-site chair massage therapy program was provided to reduce anxiety levels of 18 employees in a downsizing organization. 15 control group subjects participated in break therapy. Subjects' stress levels were measured with the State-Trait Anxiety Inventory, which was administered twice during pretest, post-test, and delayed post-test to achieve stable measures.
Results: Significant reductions in anxiety levels were found for the massage group.

AROMATHERAPY

Buckle J (1993). Aromatherapy. *Nursing Times* **89:32–35**

Method: A randomized, double-blind trial was conducted on two essential oils of two different species of lavender, topically applied on post-cardiotomy patients. The emotional and behavioral stress levels of 28 patients were evaluated pre- and post-treatment on two consecutive days.
Results: The therapeutic effects of the two lavenders appeared to be different: one was almost twice as effective as the other, thereby disproving the hypothesis that aromatherapy, using topical application of essential oils, is effective purely because of touch, massage or placebo.

Burnett KM, Solterbeck LA, Strapp CM (2004). Scent and mood state following an anxiety-provoking task. *Psychological Reports* **95:707–722**

Method: The purpose of this study was to assess the effects of water, lavender, or rosemary scent on physiology and mood state following an anxiety-provoking task. The non-smoking participants, ages 18–30 years, included 42 women and 31 men who reported demographic information, and measures of external temperature and heart rate were taken prior to introduction of an anxiety-eliciting task and exposure to lavender, rosemary, or water scents. Following the task, participants completed the Profile of Mood States to assess mood, and temperature and heart rate were reassessed. Participants rated the pleasantness of the scent received.
Results: When pleasantness ratings of scent were covaried, physiological changes in temperature and heart rate did not differ based on scent exposure, but mood ratings differed by scent condition. Participants in the rosemary condition scored higher on measures of tension-anxiety and confusion-bewilderment relative to the lavender and control conditions. The lavender and control conditions showed higher mean vigor-activity ratings relative to

the rosemary group, while both rosemary and lavender scents were associated with lower mean ratings on the fatigue-inertia subscale, relative to the control group.

Diego M, Jones NA, Field T, et al (1998). Aromatherapy positively affects mood, EEG patterns of alertness and math computations. *International Journal of Neuroscience* **96:217–224**

Method: EEG activity, alertness, mood and cortisol levels were assessed in 40 adults given 3 minutes of aromatherapy using two aromas; lavender (considered a relaxing odor) or rosemary (considered a stimulating odor). Participants were also given simple math computations before and after the therapy.
Results: The lavender group showed increased beta power suggesting increased drowsiness, they had less depressed mood (POMS) and reported feeling more relaxed and they performed the math computations faster and more accurately following aromatherapy. The rosemary group, on the other hand, showed decreased frontal alpha and beta power, suggesting increased alertness. They also had lower state anxiety scores, reported feeling more relaxed and alert and they were only faster, not more accurate, at completing the math computations after the aromatherapy session.

Fernandez M, Hernandez-Reif M, Field T, et al (2004). EEG during lavender and rosemary exposure in infants of depressed and non-depressed mothers. *British Journal of Psychology* **27:91–100**

Method: This study investigated whether exposure to pleasant odors would change electroencephalographic (EEG) activity in infants of depressed and non-depressed mothers. 20 newborns were exposed to a 10% v/v concentration of rosemary oil or lavender oil and their EEG was recorded for 2 minutes each at baseline and during odor exposure. Group inclusion (depressed vs non-depressed) was based on mothers' CES-D depression scores.
Results: Results revealed that the groups did not differ at baseline and that the two odors did not differentially affect the EEG. However, the infants of depressed mothers showed increased relative left frontal EEG activation while infants of non-depressed mothers showed increased relative right frontal EEG activation from baseline to the odor exposure phase. Relative left frontal EEG activation has been associated with an approaching pattern of behavior and response to positive stimuli, while relative right frontal EEG activation has been associated with a withdrawing pattern of behavior and response to negative stimuli. These results suggest that infants of depressed and non-depressed mothers respond differently to odors.

Goubet N, Rattaz C, Pierrat V, et al (2003). Olfactory experience mediates response to pain in preterm newborns. *Developmental Psychobiology* **42:171–180**

Method: This study assessed the effects of a familiar odor during routine blood draws in healthy preterm newborns. Infants were observed as they were undergoing either a capillary puncture on the heel (heelstick) or a venous puncture on the hand. During the procedure, one-third of the infants were presented with an odor they had been familiarized with prior to the procedure, one-third of the infants were presented with an odor they had not been previously exposed to, and one-third were presented with no odor.

Results: Heelsticks elicited more behavioral distress than venipunctures. Infants who were presented with a familiar odor during venipuncture showed no significant increase in crying and grimacing during the procedure compared to baseline levels. By comparison, infants presented with an unfamiliar odor or with no odor either during the heelstick or the venipuncture had a significant increase in crying and grimacing. When the pain was milder, i.e., during a venipuncture, and a familiar odor was presented, infants showed little to no crying.

Kim MJ, Nam ES, Paik SI (2005). The effects of aromatherapy on pain, depression, and life satisfaction of arthritis patients. *Taehan Kanho Hakhow Chi* **35:186–194**

Method: The purpose of this study was to investigate the effect of aromatherapy on pain, depression, and feelings of satisfaction in life of arthritis patients. This study used a quasi-experimental design with a non-equivalent control group, pre- and post-test. The sample consisted of 40 patients. The essential oils used were lavender, marjoram, eucalyptus, rosemary, and peppermint blended in proportions of 2:1:2:1:1. They were mixed with a carrier oil composed of almond (45%), apricot (45%), and jojoba oil (10%) and they were diluted to 1.5% after blending.

Results: Aromatherapy significantly decreased both the pain score and the depression score of the experimental group compared with the control group.

ARTHRITIS

Field T, Hernandez-Reif M, Seligman S, et al (1997). Juvenile rheumatoid arthritis: benefits from massage therapy. *Journal of Pediatric Psychology* **22:607–617**

Method: Children with mild to moderate juvenile rheumatoid arthritis were massaged by their parents 15 minutes a day for 30 days (and a control group engaged in relaxation therapy).

Results: The children's anxiety and stress hormone (cortisol) levels were immediately decreased by the massage, and over the 30-day period their pain decreased on self-reports, parent reports, and their physician's assessment of pain (both the incidence and severity) and pain-limiting activities.

Yurtkuran M, Kocagil T (1999). TENS, electropuncture and ice massage: comparison of treatment for osteoarthritis of the knee. *American Journal of Acupuncture* **27:133–140**

Method: The purpose of this study was to compare the effectiveness of transcutaneous electrical nerve stimulation (TENS), electroacupuncture (EA), and ice massage with placebo treatment for the treatment of pain. Subjects (n = 100) diagnosed with osteoarthritis (OA) of the knee were treated with these modalities. The parameters for evaluating the effectiveness of treatment included pain at rest, stiffness, 50 foot walking time, quadriceps muscle strength, and knee flexion degree.

Results: The results showed (a) that all three methods could be effective in decreasing not only pain but also the objective parameters in a short period of time; and (b) that the treatment results in TENS, EA and ice massage were superior to placebo.

ASTHMA

Field T, Henteleff T, Hernandez-Reif M, et al (1997). Children with asthma have improved pulmonary functions after massage therapy. *Journal of Pediatrics* **132:854–858**

Method: Thirty-two children with asthma (16 4- to 8-year-olds and 16 9- to 14-year-olds) were randomly assigned to receive either massage therapy or relaxation therapy. The children's parents were taught to provide one therapy or the other for 20 minutes before bedtime each night for 30 days.

Results: The younger children who received massage therapy showed an immediate decrease in behavioral anxiety and cortisol levels after massage. Also, their attitude toward asthma and their peak air flow and other pulmonary functions improved over the course of the study. The older children who received massage therapy reported lower anxiety after the massage. Their attitude toward asthma also improved over the study, but only one measure of pulmonary function (forced expiratory flow 25% to 75%) improved. The reason for the smaller therapeutic benefit in the older children is unknown; however, it appears that daily massage improves airway caliber and control of asthma.

ATTENTION DEFICIT HYPERACTIVITY DISORDER

Field T, Quintino O, Hernandez-Reif M, et al (1998). Adolescents with attention deficit hyperactivity disorder benefit from massage therapy. *Adolescence* **33:103–108**

Method: Twenty-eight adolescents with attention deficit hyperactivity disorder were provided with either massage therapy or relaxation therapy for 10 consecutive school days.

Results: The massage therapy group, but not the relaxation therapy group, rated themselves as happier and observers rated them as fidgeting less following the sessions. After the 2-week period, their teachers reported more time on task and assigned them lower hyperactivity scores based on classroom behavior.

Hernandez-Reif M, Field T, Thimas E (2001). Attention deficit hyperactivity disorder: benefits from Tai Chi. *Journal of Bodywork and Movement Therapies* **5:120–123**

Method: Thirteen adolescents with attention deficit hyperactivity disorder (ADHD) participated in Tai Chi classes twice a week for 5 weeks. Teachers rated the children's behavior on the Conners Scale during the baseline period, after the 5-week Tai Chi session period and 2 weeks later.

Results: After the 10 Tai Chi sessions the adolescents displayed less anxiety, improved conduct, less daydreaming behaviors, less inappropriate emotions, and less hyperactivity. These improved scores persisted over the 2-week follow up (no Tai Chi period).

Khilnani S, Field T, Hernandez-Reif M, et al (2003). Massage therapy improves mood and behavior of students with attention-deficit/hyperactivity disorder. *Adolescence* **38:623–638**

Method: The present study involved 30 children and adolescents between the ages of 7 and 18 (mean age = 13) diagnosed with attention-deficit/hyperactivity disorder (ADHD). The children were randomly assigned to a wait-list control and a massage group. The latter group received massage therapy for 20 minutes twice per week over the course of 1 month.

Results: Mood state improved for the massage but not the control group based on smiley face and thermometer scales. The massage group also improved in classroom behavior in the areas of the Conners Teacher Rating Scales on anxiety, daydreaming and hyperactivity. The wait-list control group did not show these gains. In sum, the results revealed that massage therapy benefited children and adolescents with ADHD by improving short-term mood state and longer-term classroom behavior.

AUTISM

Escalona A, Field T, Singer-Strunk R, et al (2001). Improvements in the behavior of children with autism. *Journal of Autism and Developmental Disorders* **31:513–516**

Method: Twenty children with autism ranging in age from 3 to 6 years were randomly assigned to massage therapy and reading attention control groups. Parents in the massage therapy group were trained by a massage therapist to massage their children for 15 minutes prior to bedtime every night for 1 month while the parents of the attention control group read Dr Seuss stories to their children on the same time schedule. Teacher and Parent scales, classroom and playground observations and sleep diaries were used to assess the effects of therapy on various behaviors including hyperactivity, stereotypical and off-task behavior, as well as sleep problems.

Results: Results suggested that the children in the massage group exhibited less stereotypic behavior and showed more on-task and social relatedness behavior during play observations at school, and they experienced fewer sleep problems at home.

Field T, Lasko D, Mundy P, et al (1986). Autistic children's attentiveness and responsivity improved after touch therapy. *Journal of Autism and Developmental Disorders* **27:329–334**

Method: This study investigated the effects of touch therapy on three problems commonly associated with autism, including inattentiveness (off-task behavior), touch aversion, and withdrawal.

Results: Results showed that touch aversion decreased in both the touch therapy and the touch control group, off-task behavior decreased in both groups, orienting to irrelevant sounds decreased in both groups, but significantly more in the touch therapy group, and stereotypic behaviors decreased in both groups but significantly more in the touch therapy group.

BEHAVIOR PROBLEMS

Escalona A, Field T, Cullen C, et al. In review Behavior problem preschool children benefit from massage therapy. *Early Child Development and Care*

Method: Twenty preschool children with behavior problems were randomly assigned to a massage group or a story-reading attention control group. The sessions occurred for 15-minutes twice a week for a month. Pre- and post-session ratings were made on the first and last days of the study by teachers who were blind to the child's group assignment.

Results: These revealed that the children in the massage therapy group: (1) were more drowsy, less active, less talkative and had lower anxiety levels after the sessions; and (2) were less anxious and more cooperative by the end of the study.

BLOOD FLOW

Agarwal KN, Gupta A, Pushkarna R, et al (2000). Effects of massage & use of oil on growth, blood flow & sleep pattern in infants. *Indian Journal of Medical Research* **112:212–217**

Method: This study investigated whether massage oils commonly used for infant massage were beneficial. 125 full-term healthy infants were randomly assigned to five groups: (i) herbal oil, (ii) sesame oil, (iii) mustard oil, or (iv) mineral oil for massage daily for 4 weeks. The fifth group did not receive massage and served as control.

Results: Massage improved the weight, length, and midarm and midleg circumferences as compared to infants without massage. The femoral artery blood velocity, diameter and flow also improved, as did their sleep.

Hovind H, Nielsen SL (1974). Effect of massage on blood flow in skeletal muscle. *Scandinavian Journal of Rehabilitation Medicine* 6:74–77

Method: Skeletal muscle blood flow was measured before, during and after short application of different forms of massage using the local Xenon washout method for determination of blood flow.

Results: During maneuvers with tapotement (pounding) an increase in blood flow comparable to exercise hyperemia was observed, and this increase was ascribed to repetitive contractions. During and after petrissage (kneading) the tissue perfusion did not change significantly.

Shoemaker JK, Tidus PM, Mader R (1997). Failure of manual massage to alter limb blood flow: measures by Doppler ultrasound. *Medicine and Science in Sports and Exercise* 1:610–614

Method: The ability of manual massage to alter muscle blood flow through three types of massage treatments in a small (forearm) and a large (quadriceps) muscle mass was tested in 10 healthy individuals. A certified massage therapist administered effleurage, petrissage, and tapotement treatments to the forearm flexors (small muscle mass) and quadriceps (large muscle mass) muscle groups in a counterbalanced manner. Limb blood flow was determined from mean blood velocity (MBV) (pulsed Doppler) and vessel diameter (echo Doppler). MBV values were obtained from the continuous data sets prior to treatment, and at 5, 10, and 20 s and 5 min following the onset of massage. Arterial diameters were measured immediately prior to and following the massage treatments; these values were not different and were averaged for the blood flow calculations.

Results: The MBV and blood flows for brachial and femoral arteries, respectively, were not altered by any of the massage treatments in either the forearm or quadriceps muscle groups. Mild voluntary handgrip and knee extension contractions resulted in peak blood velocities and blood flow for brachial and femoral arteries, respectively, which were significantly elevated from rest. The results indicated that manual massage did not elevate muscle blood flow irrespective of massage type or the muscle mass receiving the treatment.

BLOOD PRESSURE

Kurosawa M, Lundeberg T, Agren G, et al (1995). Massage-like stroking of the abdomen lowers blood pressure in anesthetized rats: influence of oxytocin. *Journal of the Autonomic Nervous System* 56:26–30

Method: The aim of this study was to determine how massage-like stroking of the abdomen in rats influences blood pressure. The ventral and/or lateral sides of the abdomen were stroked in anesthetized, artificially ventilated rats. Arterial blood pressure was recorded with a pressure transducer via catheter in the carotid artery.

Results: Stroking of the ventral or both ventral and lateral sides of the abdomen for 1 minute caused a marked decrease in blood pressure. After cessation of the stimulation blood pressure returned to the control level within 1 minute. Stroking only the lateral sides of the abdomen elicited a significantly smaller decrease in blood pressure than stroking the ventral side. This effect did not involve oxytocin.

BREAST CANCER

Hernandez-Reif M, Ironson G, Field T, et al (2004). Breast cancer patients have improved immune functions following massage therapy. *Journal of Psychosomatic Research* **57(1):45–52**

Method: Thirty-four women (mean age = 53) diagnosed with Stage I or II breast cancer were randomly assigned post-surgery to a massage therapy group (to receive 30-minute massages three times per week for 5 weeks) or a standard treatment control group. On the first and last day of the study, the women were assessed on (1) immediate effects measures of anxiety, depressed mood, and vigor, and (2) longer-term effects on depression, anxiety and hostility, functioning, body image and avoidant versus intrusive coping style, in addition to urinary catecholamines (norepinephrine, epinephrine, and dopamine), and serotonin levels. A subset of 27 women (n = 15 massage) had blood drawn to assay immune measures. The immediate massage therapy effects included reduced anxiety, depressed mood, and anger. The longer-term massage effects included reduced depression and hostility, increased urinary dopamine, serotonin values, natural killer cell number and lymphocytes.
Results: Avoidance coping was associated with greater NK cell number and intrusive coping with lower dopamine levels. Women with stage I and II breast cancer may benefit from thrice-weekly massage therapy for reducing depressed mood, anxiety and anger and for enhancing dopamine, serotonin and natural killer cell number and lymphocytes.

Hernandez-Reif M, Field T, Ironson G, et al (2005). Natural killer cells and lymphocytes increase in women with breast cancer following massage therapy. *International Journal of Neuroscience* **115(4):495–510**

Method: Women diagnosed with breast cancer received massage therapy or practiced progressive muscle relaxation (PMR) for 30-minute sessions three times a week for 5 weeks, or received standard treatment. The massage therapy and relaxation groups reported less depressed mood, anxiety and pain immediately after their first and last sessions. By the end of the study, however, only the massage therapy group reported being less depressed and less angry and having more vigor. Dopamine levels, natural killer cells and lymphocytes also increased from the first to the last day of the study for the massage therapy group. These findings highlight the benefit of these complementary therapies, most particularly massage therapy, for women with breast cancer.

BREASTFEEDING

Foda MI, Kawashima T, Nakamura S, et al (2004). Composition of milk obtained from unmassaged versus massaged breasts of lactating mothers. *Journal of Pediatric Gastroenterology and Nutrition* **38:484–487**

Method: Milk samples were obtained immediately before and after massage from healthy, exclusively breastfeeding Japanese mothers at two different periods of lactation, one <3 months, the other >3 months after parturition. Lipids, whey protein, casein, lactose, ash, and total solids in milk were measured in milk samples. The gross energy content of milk was estimated.

Results: Breast massage significantly increased lipids in the late lactating period but not in the early lactating period. In the early lactating period casein was increased by breast massage but was not significantly affected in the late lactating period. Breast massage caused a significant increase in total solids from the first day to 11 months post-partum. The gross energy in the late lactating period was significantly increased by breast massage but not in the early lactating period. Lactose was not significantly changed by breast massage.

Jones E, Dimmock PW, Spencer SA (2001). A randomised controlled trial to compare methods of milk expression after preterm delivery. Archives of Disease in Childhood. *Fetal and Neonatal Edition* **85(2):F91–F95**

Method: Primary: to compare sequential and simultaneous breast pumping on volume of milk expressed and its fat content. Secondary: to measure the effect of breast massage on milk volume and fat content.

Design: Sequential randomized controlled trial.

Setting: Neonatal intensive care unit, North Staffordshire Hospital NHS Trust.

Subjects: Data on 36 women were analyzed; 19 women used simultaneous pumping and 17 used sequential pumping.

Interventions: Women were randomly allocated to use either simultaneous (both breasts simultaneously) or sequential (one breast then the other) milk expression. Stratification was used to ensure that the groups were balanced for parity and gestation. A crossover design was used for massage, with patients acting as their own controls. Women were randomly allocated to receive either massage or non-massage first.

Main outcome measures: Volume of milk expressed per expression and its fat content (estimated by the creamatocrit method).

Results: Milk yield per expression was: sequential pumping with no massage, 51.32 g (95% confidence interval (CI) 56.57–46.07); sequential pumping with massage, 78.71 g (95% CI 85.19–72.24); simultaneous pumping with no massage, 87.69 g (95% CI 96.80–78.57); simultaneous pumping with massage,

125.08 g (95% CI 140.43–109.74). The fat concentration in the milk was not affected by the increase in volume achieved by the interventions.

Conclusions: The results are unequivocal and show that simultaneous pumping is more effective at producing milk than sequential pumping and that breast massage has an additive effect, improving milk production in both groups. As frequent and efficient milk removal is essential for continued production of milk, mothers of preterm infants wishing to express milk for their sick babies should be taught these techniques.

BREAST MASSAGE

Yokoyama Y, Ueda T, Irahara M, et al (1994). Releases of oxytocin and pro-lactin during breast massage and suckling in puerperal women. *European Journal of Obstetrics, Gynecology & Reproductive Biology* **53:17–20**

Method: The responses of prolactin and oxytocin to suckling and breast massage were examined in lactating women.

Results: The suckling group showed an increase in frequency of pulsatile release of oxytocin and an increase in the plasma prolactin level. In contrast, the breast massage group showed a significant, but not a pulsatile increase in the plasma oxytocin level and no increase in the plasma prolactin level. These findings suggest that suckling causes both milk production and milk ejection, while breast massage causes only ejection of milk already stored, and that prolactin release is not related to an increase of the oxytocin level itself, but to its pulsatile release.

BULIMIA

Field T, Schanberg S, Kuhn C, et al (1998). Bulimic adolescents benefit from massage therapy. *Adolescence* **33:555–563**

Method: Twenty-four female adolescent bulimic inpatients were randomly assigned to a massage therapy or a standard treatment (control) group.

Results: The massaged patients showed immediate reductions in anxiety and depression (both self-report and behavior observation). In addition, by the last day of the therapy, they had lower depression scores, lower cortisol (stress) levels, higher dopamine levels, and showed improvement on several other psychological and behavioral measures.

BURNS

Field T, Peck M, Krugman S, et al (1998). Burn injuries benefit from massage therapy. *Journal of Burn Care and Rehabilitation* **19:241–244**

Method: Twenty-eight adult patients with burns were randomly assigned before debridement to either a massage therapy group or a standard treatment control group.

Results: State anxiety and cortisol levels decreased, and behavior ratings of state, activity, vocalizations, and anxiety improved after the massage therapy sessions on the first and last days of treatment. Longer-term effects were also significantly greater for the massage therapy group including decreases in depression and anger, and decreased pain on the McGill Pain Questionnaire, Present Pain Intensity Scale, and Visual Analog Scale. Although the underlying mechanisms are not known, these data suggest that debridement sessions were less painful after the massage therapy sessions due to a reduction in anxiety, and that the clinical course was probably enhanced as a result of a reduction in pain, anger, and depression.

Field T, Peck M, Hernandez-Reif M, et al (2000). Postburn itching, pain, and psychological symptoms are reduced with massage therapy. *Journal of Burn Care & Rehabilitation* **21:189–193**

Method: Twenty patients with burn injuries were randomly assigned to a massage therapy or a standard treatment control group during the remodeling phase of wound healing. The massage therapy group received a 30-minute massage with cocoa butter to a closed, moderate-sized scar tissue area twice a week for 5 weeks.

Results: The massage therapy group reported reduced itching, pain, and anxiety and improved mood immediately after the first and last therapy sessions, and their ratings on these measures improved from the first day to the last day of the study.

Hernandez-Reif M, Field T, Largie S, et al (2001). Children's distress during burn treatment is reduced by massage therapy. *Journal of Burn Care and Rehabilitation* **22:191–195**

Method: Before dressing changes, 24 young children (mean age = 2.5 years) hospitalized for severe burns received standard dressing care or massage therapy in addition to standard dressing care. The massage therapy was conducted to body parts that were not burned.

Results: During the dressing change, the children who received massage therapy showed minimal distress behaviors and no increase in movement other than torso movement. In contrast, the children who did not receive massage therapy responded to the dressing change procedure with increased facial grimacing, torso movement, crying, leg movement and reaching out. Nurses also reported greater ease in completing the dressing change procedure for the children in the massage therapy group. These findings suggest that massage therapy attenuates young children's distress responses to aversive medical procedures and facilitates dressing changes.

CANCER

Ferrell-Torry AT, Glick OJ (1973). The use of therapeutic massage as a nursing intervention to modify anxiety and the perception of cancer pain. *Cancer Nursing* **16:93–101**

Method: The purpose of this exploratory study was to examine the effects of therapeutic massage (consisting of effleurage, petrissage, and myofascial trigger point therapy) on pain perception, anxiety, and relaxation levels in hospitalized patients experiencing significant cancer pain. Thirty minutes of therapeutic massage were administered on two consecutive evenings to nine hospitalized males diagnosed with cancer and experiencing cancer pain. The subjects' self-reports of pain and relaxation (measured by Visual Analog Scales) as well as anxiety (measured by the Spielberger State Anxiety Inventory) were recorded before and immediately after the intervention. Heart rate, respiratory rate, and blood pressure were obtained before, immediately after and 10 minutes after the massage intervention.

Results: Massage therapy significantly reduced the subjects' level of pain perception (average = 60%) and anxiety (average = 24%) while enhancing their feelings of relaxation by an average of 58%. In addition to these subjective measures, all physiological measures (heart rate, respiratory rate, and blood pressure) tended to decrease from baseline, providing further indication of relaxation. In conclusion, although the exact mechanism is not known, therapeutic massage is a beneficial nursing intervention that promotes relaxation and alleviates the perception of pain and anxiety in hospitalized cancer patients.

Forchuk C, Baruth P, Prendergast M, et al (2004). Postoperative arm massage: a support for women with lymph node dissection. *Cancer Nursing* **27:25–33**

Method: To evaluate the usefulness of arm massage from a significant other following lymph node dissection surgery.

Design: Randomized clinical trial with a pretest–post-test design. Data were collected prior to surgery, within 24 hours post surgery, within 10 to 14 days post surgery, and 4 months post surgery.

Sample: 59 women, aged 21 to 78 undergoing lymph node dissection surgery and who had a significant other with them during the postoperative period. Subjects were randomly assigned to intervention and control groups. Subjects' significant others in the intervention group were first taught, then performed arm massage as a postoperative support measure.

Research main variables: Variables included postoperative pain, family strengths and stressors, range of motion, and health related costs.

Results: Participants reported a reduction in pain in the immediate postoperative period and better shoulder function. Arm massage decreased pain and discomfort related to surgery, and promoted a sense of closeness and support amongst subjects and their significant other.

Implication for nursing practice: Postoperative massage therapy for women with lymph node dissection provided therapeutic benefits for patients and their significant other. Nurses can offer effective alternative interventions along with standard procedures in promoting optimal health.

Goodfellow LM (2003). The effects of therapeutic back massage on psychophysiologic variables and immune function in spouses of patients with cancer. *Nursing Research* **52:318–328**

Method: Spouses of patients with cancer are at risk for stress-related disorders and may experience a reduction in immune function. Therapeutic back massage (TBM) has been shown to enhance relaxation and thus, may reduce stress associated with caring for an ill partner.

Objectives: To determine if TBM's influences on psychosocial, physiologic, and immune function variables in spouses of patients with cancer, and explore the relationships between psychosocial variables and immune function in spouses of patients with cancer. This group experimental design measured the effects of a 20-minute TBM at three time points (preintervention, immediately postintervention, 20 minutes postintervention) on spouses of patients with cancer (n = 42) randomly assigned to either the experimental or control group. The major dependent variables including natural killer cell activity (NKCA), heart rate, systolic and diastolic blood pressure, mood, and perceived stress were measured at the three time points to examine the effects of TBM. Data collected on measures of mood and perceived stress were correlated with NKCA to examine their relationships. Prior to hypotheses testing, data collected on measures of depressive mood, loneliness, marital disruption, and health practices were also correlated with NKCA to ascertain any possible confounding variables.

Results: Two-way repeated measures analysis of variance tests determined the effects of TBM over the two postintervention time points and resulted in significant group × time interactions on mood (F [2, 40] = 14.61, p = 0.0005) and perceived stress (F [2, 40] = 28.66, p = 0.001). Significant inverse relationships were found between mood and NKCA (r = –0.41, p = 0.009, n = 42) and perceived stress and NKCA (r = –0.37, p = 0.017, n = 42).

Discussion: Findings suggest that TBM may enhance mood and reduce perceived stress in this population. Insight was gained into the psychoimmunologic relationships studied.

Grealish L, Lomasney A, Whiteman B (2000). Foot massage. A nursing intervention to modify the distressing symptoms of pain and nausea in patients hospitalized with cancer. *Cancer Nursing* **23:237–243**

Methods: This article describes the findings of an empirical study on the use of foot massage as a nursing intervention in patients hospitalized with cancer.

Results: In a sample of 87 subjects, a 10-minute foot massage (5 minutes per foot) was found to reduce perceptions of pain, nausea, and relaxation when measured with a visual analog scale.

Rexilius SJ, Mundt C, Erickson Megel M, et al (2002). Therapeutic effects of massage therapy and handling touch on caregivers of patients undergo-

ing autologous hematopoietic stem cell transplant.   *Oncology Nursing Forum* 29:E35–44

Method: This study examined the effects of massage therapy and Healing Touch on anxiety, depression, subjective caregiver burden, and fatigue experienced by caregivers of patients undergoing autologous hematopoietic stem cell transplant.
Design: Quasi-experimental repeated measures.
Setting: Oncology/hematology outpatient clinic in a large midwestern city.
Sample: 36 caregivers: 13 in the control group, 13 in the massage therapy group, and 10 in the Healing Touch group. Average age was 51.5 years; most participants were Caucasian. All caregivers completed the Beck Anxiety Inventory, the Center for Epidemiologic Studies Depression Scale, the Subjective Burden Scale, and the Multidimensional Fatigue Inventory-20 before and after treatment consisting of two 30-minute massages or Healing Touch treatments per week for 3 weeks. Caregivers in the control group received usual nursing care and a 10-minute supportive visit from one of the researchers.
Results: Results showed significant declines in anxiety scores, depression, general fatigue, reduced motivation fatigue, and emotional fatigue for individuals in the massage therapy group only.

Shin YH, Kim TI, Shin MS, et al (2004). Effect of acupressure on nausea and vomiting during chemotherapy cycle for Korean postoperative stomach cancer patients. *Cancer Nursing* 27:267–274

Method: Despite the development of effective antiemetic drugs, nausea and vomiting remain the main side-effects associated with cancer chemotherapy. The purpose of this study was to examine the effect of acupressure on emesis control in postoperative gastric cancer patients undergoing chemotherapy. Forty postoperative gastric cancer patients receiving the first cycle of chemotherapy with cisplatin and 5-Fluorouracil were divided into control and intervention groups (n = 20 each). Both groups received regular antiemesis medication; however, the intervention group received acupressure training and was instructed to perform the finger acupressure maneuver for 5 minutes on P6 (Nei-Guan) point located at 3-finger widths up from the first palmar crease, between palmaris longus and flexor carpi radialis tendons point, at least three times a day before chemotherapy and mealtimes or based on their needs. Both groups received equally frequent nursing visits and consultations, and reported nausea and vomiting using Rhode's Index of Nausea, Vomiting and Retching.
Results: We found significant differences between intervention and control groups in the severity of nausea and vomiting, the duration of nausea, and frequency of vomiting. This study suggests that acupressure on P6 point appears to be an effective adjunct maneuver in the course of emesis control.

Smith MC, Kemp J, Hemphill L, et al (2002). Outcomes of therapeutic massage for hospitalized cancer patients. *Journal of Nursing Scholarship* 34:257–262

Method: To examine the effects of therapeutic massage on perception of pain, subjective sleep quality, symptom distress, and anxiety in patients hospitalized for treatment of cancer.

Organizing construct: Rogers' Science of Unitary Human Beings and Watson's theory of human caring. Quasi-experimental. The sample consisted of 41 patients admitted to the oncology unit at a large urban medical center in the United States for chemotherapy or radiation therapy. Twenty participants received therapeutic massage and 21 received the control therapy, nurse interaction. The outcome variables were measured on admission and at the end of 1 week via the following instruments: a Numerical Rating Scale for pain intensity and Likert-type scale for distress from pain; The Verran and Snyder-Halpern Sleep Scale, McCorkle and Young's Symptom Distress Scale, and the Spielberger State Anxiety Inventory. ANOVA and t tests were used to analyze between and within group differences in mean scores and main effects on outcome variables.

Results: Mean scores for pain, sleep quality, symptom distress, and anxiety improved from baseline for the subjects who received therapeutic massage; only anxiety improved from baseline for participants in the comparison group. Statistically significant interactions were found for pain, symptom distress, and sleep. Sleep improved only slightly for the participants receiving massage, but it deteriorated significantly for those in the control group. The findings support the potential for massage as a nursing therapeutic for cancer patients receiving chemotherapy or radiation therapy.

Soden K, Vincent K, Craske S, et al (2004). A randomized controlled trial of aromatherapy massage in a hospice setting. *Palliative Medicine* 18:87–92

Method: Research suggests that patients with cancer, particularly in the palliative care setting, are increasingly using aromatherapy and massage. There is good evidence that these therapies may be helpful for anxiety reduction for short periods, but few studies have looked at the longer term effects. This study was designed to compare the effects of 4-week courses of aromatherapy massage and massage alone on physical and psychological symptoms in patients with advanced cancer. Forty-two patients were randomly allocated to receive weekly massages with lavender essential oil and an inert carrier oil (aromatherapy group), an inert carrier oil only (massage group) or no intervention. Outcome measures included a Visual Analog Scale (VAS) of pain intensity, the Verran and Snyder-Halpern (VSH) sleep scale, the Hospital Anxiety and Depression (HAD) scale and the Rotterdam Symptom Checklist (RSCL).

Results: We were unable to demonstrate any significant long-term benefits of aromatherapy or massage in terms of improving pain control, anxiety or quality of life. Sleep scores improved significantly in both the massage and the combined massage (aromatherapy and massage) groups. There were also statistically significant reductions in depression scores in the massage group. In this study of patients with advanced cancer, the addition of lavender essential oil did not appear to increase the beneficial effects of massage. Our results do suggest, however, that patients with high levels of psychological distress respond best to these therapies.

Stephenson NL, Weinrich SP, Tavakoli AS (2000). The effects of foot reflexology on anxiety and pain in patients with breast and lung cancer. *Oncology Nursing Forum* **27:67–72**

Method: To test the effects of foot reflexology on anxiety and pain in patients with breast and lung cancer.
Results: Following the foot reflexology intervention, patients with breast and lung cancer experienced a significant decrease in anxiety. One of three pain measures showed that patients with breast cancer experienced a significant decrease in pain.

Wilkie DJ, Kampbell J, Cutshall S, et al (2000). Effects of massage on pain intensity, analgesics and quality of life in patients with cancer pain: a pilot study of a randomized clinical trial conducted within hospice care delivery. *Hospice Journal* **15:31–53**

Method: This randomized controlled clinical trial examined the effects of massage on perceived pain intensity, prescribed morphine, hospital admissions, and quality of life. Of 173 hospice patients with terminal cancer, 29 (aged 30–85 yrs) completed the 3-week pilot study. 14 subjects (controls) were assigned to usual hospice care and 15 subjects were assigned to usual hospice care with massage interventions consisting of four twice-weekly massages. Baseline and outcome measurements were obtained before the 1st and after the 4th massages.
Results: Pain intensity, pulse rate, and respiratory rate were significantly reduced immediately after the massages. At study entry, the massage group reported higher pain intensity which decreased by 42% compared to a 25% reduction in the control group.

CARDIOVASCULAR

Boone T, Cooper R (1995). The effect of massage on oxygen consumption at rest. *American Journal of Chinese Medicine* **23:37–41**

Method: This study determined the effect of massage on oxygen consumption at rest. Ten healthy, adult males (mean age = 28 years) volunteered to serve as subjects. During the Control Session, each subject was placed in the supine position on a massage table to remain motionless for 30 minutes. During the Treatment Session, each subject received a 30-minute sports massage of the lower extremities. Oxygen consumption was determined via the Beckman

Metabolic Measurement Chart, which was upgraded to estimate cardiac output using the CO_2 rebreathing (equilibrium) method.

Results: The subjects' oxygen consumption did not change with the massage. Also, there were no significant differences in heart rate, stroke volume, cardiac output, and arteriovenous oxygen difference during the massage. These findings indicate that massaging the lower extremities results in neither an increase nor a decrease in the subjects' expenditure of energy at rest.

Boone T, Tanner M, Radosevich A (2001). Effects of a 10-minute back rub on cardiovascular responses in healthy subjects. *American Journal of Chinese Medicine* 29:47–52

Method: This study determined the cardiovascular responses to a 10-minute back rub. Twelve healthy, college-age males and females volunteered to participate as subjects. The subjects were assessed for 10 minutes lying on one side on a massage table. During the treatment period, a back rub was administered. Oxygen consumption and cardiac output were measured.

Results: The central and peripheral components of oxygen consumption were changed and cardiac output decreased. These results indicate that the back rub was effective in inducing relaxation.

Delaney JP, Leong KS, Watkins A, et al (2002). The short-term effects of myofascial trigger point massage therapy on cardiac autonomic tone in healthy subjects. *Journal of Advanced Nursing* 37:364–371

Method: This study investigated the effects of myofascial trigger-point massage therapy to the head, neck and shoulder areas on cardiac autonomic tone. The study involved 30 healthy subjects (16 female and 14 male), aged 32. A 5-minute cardiac interbeat interval recording, systolic and diastolic blood pressure and subjective self-evaluations of muscle tension and emotional state were taken before and after intervention.

Results: Following myofascial trigger-point massage therapy there was a significant decrease in heart rate, systolic blood pressure and diastolic blood pressure. Analysis of heart rate variability revealed a significant increase in parasympathetic activity following myofascial trigger-point massage therapy. Additionally both muscle tension and emotional state showed significant improvement.

McNamara ME, Burnham DC, Smith C, et al (2003). The effects of back massage before diagnostic cardiac catheterization. *Alternative Therapies in Health and Medicine* 9:50–57

Method: Admission to the hospital for a diagnostic cardiac catheterization can be perceived as a threat to one's health status. Autonomic nervous system arousal, particularly the sympathetic division, can elicit negative physiological and psychological human responses as a reaction to this threat. The purpose of this study was to measure the effects of a 20-minute back massage on the physiological and psychological human responses of patients admitted for a diagnostic cardiac catheterization. A randomized clinical trial design was used. Data were compared in a repeated measures design before massage (T1), immediately following the back massage or standard care (T2), and 10 minutes later (T3).

Setting: A large urban academic medical center.

Participants: Forty-six subjects admitted from home for a diagnostic cardiac catheterization.

Main outcome measures: Heart rate, heart rate variability, blood pressure, respiration, peripheral skin temperature, pain perception, and psychological state.

Intervention: A 20-minute back massage.

Results: There was a significant difference between subject effect for group, with a reduction in systolic blood pressure in the treatment group (F = 8.6, $p < 0.05$). In addition, main effects were noted for time for diastolic blood pressure (F = 5.44; $p < 0.006$), respiration (F = 10.6; $p < 0.005$), total Profile of Mood States score (F = 5.9; $p < 0.001$) and pain perception (F = 4.09; $p < 0.04$) in both groups.

Discussion: A 20-minute back massage appeared to reduce systolic blood pressure in patients awaiting a diagnostic cardiac catheterization, while preparatory time in the cardiac catheterization laboratory appeared to reduce diastolic blood pressure, respiration, perceived psychological distress, and pain.

CARPAL TUNNEL SYNDROME

Field T, Diego M, Cullen C, et al (2004). Carpal tunnel syndrome symptoms are lessened following massage therapy. *Journal of Bodywork and Movement Therapies* **8:9–14**

Method: The objective of this study was to determine the effectiveness of massage therapy for relieving the symptoms of carpal tunnel syndrome (CTS). Sixteen adults with CTS symptoms were randomized to a 4-week massage therapy or control group. Participants in the massage therapy group were taught a self-massage routine that was done daily at home. They were also massaged once a week by a therapist. The participants' diagnosis was based on a nerve conduction velocity test, the Phalen test, and the Tinel sign test performed by a physician. The participants were also given the State Trait Anxiety Inventory, the Profile of Mood States, a visual analog scale for pain and a test of grip strength.

Results: Participants in the massage therapy group improved on median peak latency and grip strength. They also experienced lower levels of perceived pain, anxiety, and depressed mood. The results suggest that symptoms of CTS might be relieved by a daily regimen of massage therapy.

CEREBRAL PALSY

Hernandez-Reif M, Field T, Largie S, et al (2005). Cerebral palsy symptoms in children decreased following massage therapy. *Early Child Development and Care* **175:445–456**

Method: Twenty young children (mean age = 32 months) with cerebral palsy (CP) recruited from early intervention programs received 30-minutes of massage or reading twice weekly for 12 weeks.

Results: The children receiving massage therapy showed fewer physical symptoms including reduced spasticity and less rigid muscle tone overall and in the arms and legs as well as improved fine and gross motor functioning. In addition, the massage group had improved cognition, social and dressing scores on the Developmental Profile and they showed more positive facial expressions and less limb activity during face-to-face play interactions. These findings suggest that massage therapy attenuates physical symptoms associated with CP, enhances development and should be considered as an early intervention for children with CP.

CHRONIC FATIGUE SYNDROME

Field T, Sunshine W, Hernandez-Reif M, et al (1997). Chronic fatigue syndrome: massage therapy effects on depression and somatic symptoms in chronic fatigue syndrome. *Journal of Chronic Fatigue Syndrome* **3:43–51**

Method: Twenty adults with chronic fatigue syndrome were randomly assigned to a massage therapy or a sham TENS (transcutaneous electrical nerve stimulation) control group.

Results: Immediately following the massage therapy versus the sham TENS sessions on the first and last days of the study the massage therapy group had lower depression and anxiety scores and lower cortisol levels. Longer-term effects (last day versus first day) suggested that the massage therapy versus the sham TENS group had lower depression, emotional distress and somatic symptom scores, more hours of sleep and lower epinephrine and cortisol levels.

COCAINE EXPOSURE

Wheeden A, Scafidi FA, Field T, et al (1993). Massage effects on cocaine-exposed preterm neonates. *Journal of Developmental and Behavioral Pediatrics* **14:318–322**

Method: Thirty cocaine-exposed preterm neonates (mean gestational age = 30 weeks, mean birthweight = 1212 g, mean intensive care unit duration = 18 days) were randomly assigned to a massage therapy or a control group as soon as they were considered medically stable. The treatment group (n = 15) received massages for three 15-minute periods over 3 consecutive hours for a 10-day period.

Results: Findings suggested that the massaged infants (1) averaged 28% greater weight gain per day (33 vs 26 g) although the groups did not differ on intake (calories or volume), (2) experienced fewer postnatal complications and stress behaviors than the control infants, and (3) showed more mature motor behaviors on the Brazelton examination at the end of the 10-day study period.

COGNITION (LEARNING)

Cigales M, Field T, Lundy B, et al (1997). Massage enhances recovery from habituation in normal infants. *Infant Behavior and Development* 20:29–34

Method: Four-month-old infants were given 8 minutes of massage, play, or no stimulation prior to an audiovisual habituation task.
Results: Infants who received massage showed better cognitive performance than the infants in the other two conditions.

Hart S, Field T, Hernandez-Reif M, et al (1998). Preschoolers' cognitive performance improves following massage. *Early Child Development and Care* 143:59–64

Method: Preschoolers (mean age = 4 years, 4 months) were given some scales from an intelligence test (WPPSI) before and after receiving a 15-minute massage or spending 15 minutes reading stories with an experimenter.
Results: Performance on the Block Design Scale improved following massage and accuracy was greater on the Animal Pegs Scale in the massage group.

CONSTIPATION

Bishop E, McKinnon E, Weir E, et al (2003). Reflexology in the management of encopresis and chronic constipation. *Paediatric Nursing* 15:20–21

Method: Encopresis or faecal incontinence in children is an extremely distressing condition that is usually secondary to chronic constipation/stool withholding. Traditional management with enemas may add to the child's distress. This study investigated the efficacy of treating patients with encopresis and chronic constipation with reflexology. An observational study was carried out on 50 children between 3 and 14 years of age who had a diagnosis of encopresis/chronic constipation. The children received six sessions of 30 minutes of reflexology to their feet. With the help of their parents they completed questionnaires on bowel motions and soiling patterns before, during and after the treatment. A further questionnaire was completed by parents pre- and post-treatment on their attitude towards reflexology. Forty-eight of the children completed the sessions.
Results: The number of bowel motions increased and the incidence of soiling decreased. Parents were keen to try the reflexology and were satisfied with the effect of reflexology on their child's condition. It appears that reflexology

has been an effective method of treating encopresis and constipation over a 6-week period in this cohort of patients.

CYSTIC FIBROSIS

Hernandez-Reif M, Field T, Krasnegor J, et al (1999). Children with cystic fibrosis benefit from massage therapy. *Journal of Pediatric Psychology* 24:175–181

Method: Parents massaged their children with cystic fibrosis to reduce anxiety and their children's anxiety and to improve the children's mood and peak air flow readings. Twenty children (5–12 years old) with cystic fibrosis and their parents were randomly assigned to a massage therapy or a reading control group. Parents in the treatment group were instructed and asked to conduct a 20-minute child massage every night at bedtime for 1 month. Parents in the reading control group were instructed to read for 20 minutes a night with their child for 1 month. On days 1 and 30, the parents and children answered questions relating to present anxiety levels and the children answered questions relating to mood, and their peak air flow was measured.

Results: Following the first and last massage session, the children and parents reported reduced anxiety. Mood and peak air flow readings also improved for the children in the massage therapy group.

DANCERS

Leivadi S, Hernandez-Reif M, Field T, et al (1999). Massage therapy and relaxation effects on university dance students. *Journal of Dance Medicine & Science* 3:108–112

Method: Thirty female university dancers were randomly assigned to a massage therapy or relaxation therapy group. The therapies consisted of 30-minute sessions twice a week for 5 weeks.

Results: Both groups reported less depressed mood and lowered anxiety levels. However, saliva cortisol (stress hormones) decreased only for the massage therapy group. Both groups reported less neck, shoulder, and back pain after the treatment sessions and reduced back pain across the study. However, only the massage therapy group showed increased range of motion across the study, including neck extension and shoulder abduction.

DENTAL PAIN

Ottoson D, Ekblom A, Hansson P (1981). Vibratory stimulation for the relief of pain of dental origin. *Pain* 10:37–45

Method: Vibratory stimulation was used for dental pain in 36 patients. The patients were from a clinic for dental surgery and all had suffered pain for more than 2 days from pulpal inflammation, apical periodontitis or postoperative pain following extraction of an impacted wisdom tooth. Vibration at 100 Hz was applied to various points in the facial region or the skull.

Results: All patients except three experienced an effective reduction in pain intensity. In the patients who experienced pain reduction there was usually a best point at which vibration had a greater pain alleviating effect than at other points. In 16 patients the stimulation caused a reduction in pain intensity of 75–100%; out of these, 12 patients reported a complete relief of pain.

DEPRESSION

Field T, Morrow C, Valdeon C, et al (1992). Massage reduces anxiety in child and adolescent psychiatric patients. *Journal of the American Academy of Child & Adolescent Psychiatry* **31:125–131**

Method: A 30-minute back massage was given daily for a 5-day period to 52 hospitalized children and adolescents who were depressed and had adjustment disorder.

Results: Compared with a control group who viewed relaxing videotapes, the massaged subjects were less depressed and anxious and had lower saliva cortisol levels after the massage. In addition, nurses rated the subjects as being less anxious and more cooperative on the last day of the study, and nighttime sleep increased over this period. Finally, urinary cortisol and norepinephrine levels decreased, but only for the depressed subjects.

Field T, Grizzle N, Scafidi F, et al (1996). Massage and relaxation therapies' effects on depressed adolescent mothers. *Adolescence* **31:903–911**

Method: Thirty-two depressed adolescent mothers received ten 30-minute sessions of massage therapy or relaxation therapy over a 5-week period. Subjects were randomly assigned to each group.

Results: Although both groups reported lower anxiety following their first and last therapy sessions, only the massage therapy group showed behavioral and stress hormone changes including a decrease in anxious behavior, pulse, and salivary cortisol levels. A decrease in urine cortisol levels suggested lower stress following the 5-week period for the massage therapy group.

Glover V, Onozawa K, Hodgkinson A (2002). Benefits of infant massage for mothers with postnatal depression. *Seminars in Neonatology* **7:495–500**

Method: Infant massage by the mother has been popular in many cultures, especially in India, and is growing in popularity in the West. Mothers with postnatal depression often have problems interacting with their infants.

Results: A small controlled study has shown that attending a massage class can help such mothers relate better to their babies. The mechanisms by which this is achieved are not clear but may include learning to understand their babies' cues and the release of oxytocin.

Onozawa K, Glover V, Adams D, et al (2001). Infant massage improves mother–infant interaction for mothers with postnatal depression. *Journal of Affective Disorders* **63:1–3**

Method: Thirty-four primiparous depressed mothers at 4 weeks postpartum were randomly assigned either to an infant massage class and a support group (massage group) or to a support group (control group). Each group attended five weekly sessions.

Results: The depression scores fell in both groups. However, improvement of mother–infant interactions was seen only in the massage group.

DERMATITIS

Anderson C, Lis-Balchin M, Kirk-Smith M (2000). Evaluation of massage with essential oils on childhood atopic eczema. *Phytotherapy Research* **14:452–456**

Method: Eight children, born to professional working mothers were studied to test the hypothesis that massage with essential oils (aromatherapy) used as a complementary therapy in conjunction with normal medical treatment, would help alleviate the symptoms of childhood atopic eczema. The children were randomly assigned to a massage or a massage with essential oils group. They received massage once a week by a therapist and every day by the mother over a period of 8 weeks. The preferred essential oils, chosen by the mothers for their child, from 36 commonly used aromatherapy oils, were: sweet marjoram, frankincense, German chamomile, myrrh, thyme, benzoin, spike lavender and Litsea cubeba. The treatments were evaluated by means of daily daytime irritation scores and nighttime disturbance scores, determined by the mother before and during the treatment, both over an 8-week period.

Results: The results showed a significant improvement in the eczema in the two groups of children following therapy, but there was no significant difference in improvement shown between the aromatherapy massage and massage-only group. Further studies on the essential oil massage group showed a deterioration in the eczematous condition after two further 8-week periods of therapy, following a period of rest after the initial period of contact. This may have been due to a decline in the novelty of the treatment, or, it strongly suggests possible allergic contact dermatitis provoked by the essential oils themselves.

Schachner L, Field T, Hernandez-Reif M, et al (1998). Atopic dermatitis symptoms decreased in children following massage therapy. *Pediatric Dermatology* **15:390–395**

Method: Young children with atopic dermatitis were treated with standard topical care and massage by their parents for 20 minutes daily for a 1-month period. A control group received standard topical care only.

Results: The children's affect and activity level significantly improved, and their parents' anxiety decreased immediately after the massage therapy sessions. Over the 1-month period, the parents of the massaged children reported lower anxiety levels in their children, and the children improved significantly on all clinical measures including redness, scaling, lichenification, excoriation, and pruritus. The control group only improved significantly on the scaling measure.

DIABETES

Field T, Hernandez-Reif M, LaGreca A, et al (1997). Massage therapy lowers blood glucose levels in children with diabetes mellitus. *Diabetes Spectrum* **10:237–239**

Method: Twenty diabetic children were randomly assigned to a massage therapy or relaxation therapy group. The children's parents were taught one or the other therapy and were asked to provide them for 20 minutes before bedtime each night for 30 days.

Results: The immediate effects of the massage therapy were reduced parent anxiety and depressed mood and reduced child anxiety, fidgetiness and depressed affect. Over the 30-day period compliance on insulin and food regulation improved and blood glucose levels decreased from 159 to within the normal range (121).

DOWN'S SYNDROME

Hernandez-Reif M, Field T, Bornstein J, et al. In Review Children with Down's syndrome improved in motor function and muscle tone following massage therapy. *Early Child Development and Care*

Method: Twenty-one moderate-to-high functioning young children (mean age = 2 years) with Down's syndrome receiving early intervention (PT, OT and speech therapy) were randomly assigned to also receive two ½-hour massage therapy or reading sessions (control group) per week for 2 months. On the first and last days of the study, the children were assessed on functioning using the Developmental Programming for Infants and Young Children Scale and muscle tone using a new Likert scale.

Results: Children in the massage therapy group experienced developmental gains in fine and gross motor functioning and showed less severe hypotonicity in their limbs. These findings suggest that the addition of massage therapy to an early intervention program may enhance motor and muscle functioning for children with Down's syndrome.

EEG

Field T, Ironson G, Scafidi F, et al (1996). Massage therapy reduces anxiety and enhances EEG pattern of alertness and math computations. *International Journal of Neuroscience* **86:197–205**

Method: Twenty-six adults were given a chair massage and 24 control group adults were asked to relax in the massage chair for 15 minutes, two times per week for 5 weeks. On the first and last days of the study they were monitored for EEG before, during and after the sessions. In addition, before and after the sessions they performed math computations, they completed POMS Depression and State Anxiety Scales and they provided a saliva sample for cortisol. At the beginning of the sessions they completed Life Events, Job Stress and Chronic POMS Depression Scales.

Results: The results were as follows: (1) frontal delta power increased for both groups, suggesting relaxation; (2) the massage group showed decreased frontal alpha and beta power (suggesting enhanced alertness), while the control group showed increased alpha and beta power; (3) the massage group showed increased speed and accuracy on math computations while the control group did not change; (4) anxiety levels were lower following the massage but not the control sessions, although mood state was less depressed following both the massage and control sessions; (5) salivary cortisol levels were lower following the massage but not the control sessions but only on the first day; and (6) at the end of the 5-week period depression scores were lower for both groups but job stress scores were lower only for the massage group.

ELDERLY

Field T, Hernandez-Reif M, Quintino O, et al (1998). Elder retired volunteers benefit from giving massage therapy to infants. *Journal of Applied Gerontology* **17:229–239**

Method: This exploratory within-subjects study compared the effects of elderly volunteers giving massage to infants versus receiving massage themselves. Three times a week for 3 weeks, 10 elderly volunteers received Swedish massage sessions. For another 3 weeks, three times per week, the same elderly volunteers massaged infants at a nursery school.

Results: Immediately after the first- and last-day sessions of giving massages, the elderly retired volunteers had less anxiety and depression and lower stress hormone (salivary cortisol) levels. Over the 3-week period, depression and catecholamines (norepinephrine and epinephrine) decreased and lifestyle and health improved. These effects were not as strong for the 3-week period when they received massage, possibly because the elderly retired volunteers initially felt awkward about being massaged and because they derived more satisfaction from massaging the infants.

Fraser J, Kerr JR (1993). Psychophysiological effects of back massage on elderly institutionalized patients. *Journal of Advanced Nursing* **18:238–245**

Method: Back massage was provided for elderly residents in a long-term care institution. Twenty-one residents were randomly assigned to three groups that received back massage with normal conversation, conversation only, or no intervention. Anxiety was measured prior to back massage, immediately following, and 10 minutes later, on four consecutive evenings. The Spielberger State Anxiety Inventory (STAI), electromyographic recordings (EMG), systolic blood pressure (SBP), diastolic blood pressure (DBP) and heart rate (HR) were used as measures of anxiety.

Results: With the exception of mean DBP which showed no change from pre-test to post-test and HR which increased from post-test to a delayed time interval, there was a statistically insignificant decrease in mean scores on all variables in the back massage group from pre-test to post-test and from post-test to the delayed time interval. The anxiety (STAI) score decrease was significantly greater for the back massage group versus the no intervention group.

Hartshorn K, Delage J, Field T, et al (2001). Senior citizens benefit from movement therapy. *Journal of Bodywork and Movement Therapies* 5:1–5

Method: Sixteen senior citizens participated in four 50-minute movement therapy sessions over a 2-week period and were compared to 16 senior citizens who belonged to a wait-list control group who received the movement sessions only after the end of the study.

Results: The movement therapy participants improved in their functional motion on the Tinetti scale, and specifically on the gait scale, their leg strength increased, and their leg pain significantly decreased.

ENDORPHINS

Day JA, Mason RR, Chesrown SE (1987). Effect of massage on serum level of beta-endorphin and beta-lipotropin in healthy adults. *Physical Therapy* 67:926–930

Method: The effect of massage was evaluated on the levels of endogenous opiates in peripheral venous blood. The results were based on findings from 21 healthy, adult volunteers. The volunteers were assigned randomly to either the Control Group (n = 11) that rested but received no massage or the Experimental Group (n = 10) that received a 30-minute complete back massage.

Results: No significant pre-treatment or post-treatment difference was found in blood beta-endorphin or beta-lipotropin levels between the groups. The results indicate that massage did not change the measured serum levels of beta-endorphin or beta-lipotropin in these healthy subjects without pain.

ENURESIS

Yuksek MS, Erdem AF, Atalay C, et al (2003). Acupressure versus oxybutinin in the treatment of enuresis. *Journal of International Medical Research* 31:552–556

Method: We aimed to assess the efficacy of acupressure for treating nocturnal enuresis, compared with oxybutinin. Acupressure was administered to 12 patients by their parents, who had been taught the technique. Pressure was applied at acupuncture points Gv4, Gv15, Gv20, B23, B28, B32, H7, H9, St36, Sp4, Sp6, Sp12, Ren2, Ren3, Ren6, K3 and K5. Twelve control patients received 0.4 mg/kg oxybutinin. Parents were asked to record incidences of bed-wetting and patients and/or parents completed a questionnaire 15 days and 1, 3 and 6 months after the start of treatment. Complete and partial responses after 6 months of treatment were seen in 83.3% and 16.7%, respectively, of patients treated with acupressure, and in 58.3% and 33.3%, respectively, of children who received oxybutinin.

Results: Nocturnal enuresis can be partially treated by oxybutinin but acupressure could be an alternative non-drug therapy. Acupressure has the advantages of being non-invasive, painless and cost-effective.

EXERCISE

Rodenburg JB, Steenbeek D, Schiereck P, et al (1994). Warm-up, stretching and massage diminish harmful effects of eccentric exercise. *International Journal of Sports Medicine* **15:414–419**

Method: The combination of a warm-up, stretching exercises and massage were assessed for their effects on subjective scores for delayed onset muscle soreness (DOMS) and functional and biochemical measures. Fifty people, randomly assigned to a treatment and a control group, exercised with the forearm flexors for 30 minutes. The treatment group also performed a warm-up and stretching protocol followed by forearm exercise and massage. Functional and biochemical measures were obtained before, and 1, 24, 48, 72 and 96 hours after exercise.

Results: The median values at the five post-exercise time points differed significantly for DOMS measured when the arm was extended. Significant effects for treatment were found on the maximal force, the flexion angle of the elbow and the creatine kinase activity in blood. DOMS on pressure, extension angle, and myoglobin concentration in blood did not differ between the groups. This combination of a warm-up, stretching and massage reduced some negative effects of forearm exercise, but the results were inconsistent, since some parameters were affected by the treatment whereas others were not, despite the expected efficacy of a combination of treatments.

EXTREMITIES

Wakim KG, Martin GM, Terrier JC, et al (1949). The effects of massage on the circulation in normal and paralyzed extremities. *Archives of Physical Medicine* **30:135–144**

Method: The effects of vigorous, stimulating massage and of a modified Hoffa type of deep stroking and kneading massage on the peripheral circulation in normal and diseased extremities were studied by means of the venous occlusion plethysmograph with the compensating spirometer recorder.

Results: The data obtained justify the following conclusions: (1) There is no consistent or significant average increase in total blood flow after deep stroking and kneading massage of the extremities, in normal subjects, in those with rheumatoid arthritis or in those with spastic paralysis of the extremities. (2) There is a moderate, consistent and definite increase in circulation after deep stroking and kneading massage to the extremities of subjects who have flaccid paralysis. (3) Vigorous, stimulating massage results in consistent and significant increases in the average blood flow of the massaged extremity. (4) Neither deep stroking and kneading massage nor vigorous, stimulating massage of the extremities results in consistent or significant changes in the blood flow of the contralateral unmassaged extremities.

FACIAL MASSAGE

Yamada Y, Hatayama T, Hirata T, et al (1986). A psychological effect of facial estherapy. *Tohoku Psychologica Folia* **45:6–16**

Method: Changes in emotion, level of arousal, and facial skin state were assessed in 24 female undergraduates by the use of three types of checklists.

Results: Two adjective checklists indicated that on items of both general deactivation and deactivation-sleep factors, scores were higher after the facial esthetic massage and most subjects in the experimental group showed that their facial skin state was also improved.

FIBROMYALGIA

Field T, Diego M, Cullen C, et al (2002). Fibromyalgia pain and substance P decrease and sleep improves following massage therapy. *Journal of Clinical Rheumatology* **8:72–76**

Method: To determine the effects of massage therapy versus relaxation therapy on sleep, substance P and pain in fibromyalgia patients, 24 adult fibromyalgia patients were randomly assigned to a massage therapy or relaxation therapy group. They received 30-minute treatments twice a week for 5 weeks.

Results: Both groups showed a decrease in anxiety and depressed mood immediately after the first and last therapy sessions. However, across the course of the study only the massage therapy group reported an increase in the number of sleep hours and a decrease in their sleep movements. In addition, substance P levels decreased and the patients' physicians assigned lower disease and pain ratings and rated fewer tenderpoints in the massage therapy group.

Offenbacher M, Stucki G (2000). Physical therapy in the treatment of fibromyalgia. *Scandinavian Journal of Rheumatology - Supplement* **113:78–85**

Review: Fibromyalgia is a syndrome of unknown etiology characterized by chronic widespread pain, increased tenderness to palpation and additional symptoms such as disturbed sleep, stiffness, fatigue and psychological distress. While medications mainly focus on pain reduction, physical therapy is aimed at disease consequences such as pain, fatigue, deconditioning, muscle weakness and sleep disturbances. Based on a review of current treatment options for fibromyalgia and evidence from randomized controlled trials, cardiovascular fitness training improves cardiovascular fitness, measures of pain as well as subjective energy and work capacity and physical and social activities. Based on anecdotal evidence or small observational studies, physiotherapy may reduce overloading of the muscle system, improve postural fatigue and positioning, and condition weak muscles. Massage may reduce muscle tension and may be prescribed as an adjunct with other therapies. Acupuncture may reduce pain and increase pain threshold.

Sunshine W, Field T, Schanberg S, et al (1996). Massage therapy and transcutaneous electrical stimulation effects on fibromyalgia. *Journal of Clinical Rheumatology* **2:18–22.**

Method: Thirty adult fibromyalgia syndrome subjects were randomly assigned to a massage therapy, a transcutaneous electrical stimulation (TENS), or a transcutaneous electrical stimulation no-current group (sham TENS) for 30-minute treatment sessions two times per week for 5 weeks.

Results: The massage therapy subjects reported lower anxiety and depression, and their cortisol levels were lower immediately after the therapy sessions on the first and last days of the study. The TENS group showed similar changes, but only after therapy on the last day of the study. The massage therapy group improved on the dolorimeter measure of pain. They also reported less pain the last week, less stiffness and fatigue, and fewer nights of difficult sleeping. Thus, massage therapy was the most effective therapy with these fibromyalgia patients.

Waylonis GW, Perkins RH (1994). Post-traumatic fibromyalgia. A long-term follow-up. *American Journal of Physical Medicine & Rehabilitation* **73:403–412**

Method: This report describes a follow-up study of 176 individuals seen between 1980 and 1990, in whom a diagnosis of post-traumatic fibromyalgia was made. Sixty-seven people completed a lengthy questionnaire and underwent a confirmatory physical examination using the American College of Rheumatology Criteria to confirm or deny the presence of fibromyalgia at the time of follow-up. A total of 61% noted the onset of symptoms after a motor vehicle accident, 13% after a work injury, 7% after surgery, 5% after a sports-related injury and 14% after other various traumatic events. Fifty-six of 67 individuals had 11 or more tenderpoints (average = 13.5), three had 10 tenderpoints, and seven had fewer than 10 or no tenderpoints. Study subjects were asked to compare the use of the following for the first 2 years after onset as well as the year preceding the current evaluation: biofeedback, medications, physical therapy, manipulation, massage therapy and tenderpoint injections. In addition, questions were asked regarding symptoms commonly seen in association with fibromyalgia (fatigue, sleep disturbance, etc.).

Results: There was a dramatic reduction in the use of all forms of physical treatments. 54% continued to use over-the-counter pain medications, and 39% were on antidepressants. 85% of the patients continued to have significant symptoms and clinical evidence of fibromyalgia.

GASTROINTESTINAL MOTILITY

Chen LL, Hsu SF, Wang MH, et al (2003). Use of acupressure to improve gastrointestinal motility in women after trans-abdominal hysterectomy. *American Journal of Chinese Medicine* 31:781–790

Method: The purpose of this study was to evaluate the effectiveness of acupressure on gastrointestinal (GI) motility in women after transabdominal hysterectomy (TAH). Patients were randomly assigned to two groups of 21 and 20 patients each. The experimental group received acupressure for 3 minutes at each of three meridian points: Neiguan (PC-6), Zusanli (ST-36) and Sanyinjiao (SP-6). The control group received 3 minutes of acupressure on sham points. Acupressure was performed twice a day. A questionnaire was used to determine patients' satisfaction prior to and after afternoon acupressure. GI contractions were measured with a multifunctional stethoscope before and after acupressure.

Results: Acupressure of these three meridian points significantly ($p < 0.05$) increased GI motility in the experimental group, but there was little change in the control group ($p > 0.05$). Our conclusions are that non-invasive acupressure of these meridian points can significantly improve GI motility and can be incorporated into the technical curriculum and clinical education program of nursing schools. Patients and their family members can be taught to continue this procedure at home to enhance GI motility in patients who have undergone TAH.

GROWTH

Pauk J, Kuhn C, Field T, et al (1986). Positive effects of tactile versus kinesthetic or vestibular stimulation on neuroendocrine and ODC activity in maternally deprived rat pups. *Life Science* 39:2081–2087

Method: Previous studies in our laboratory have shown that even short-term separation of preweanling rat pups from the mother produces adverse effects on the pup. These include alterations in ornithine decarboxylase activity and in the secretion of growth hormone and corticosterone. The present study demonstrated that while intermittent heavy stroking effectively reversed or prevented all the changes associated with maternal deprivation, neither kinesthetic nor vestibular stimulation affected these responses.

Results: The results verify earlier findings from this laboratory indicating that tactile interactions between rat pups and their mother modulate pup physiology and provide experimental support for the hypothesized effects of tactile stimulation on early infant development.

Schanberg S (1995). Genetic basis for touch effects. In: Field T (ed.) Touch in early development. *Lawrence Erlbaum Associates, Inc., Hillsdale*

Data from the rat model suggest that a gene for growth needs to be triggered by touch for growth to occur.

H–REFLEX

Morelli M, Seaborne DE, Sullivan SJ (1991). H-reflex modulation during manual muscle massage of human triceps surae. *Archives of Physical Medicine & Rehabilitation* **72:915–919**

Method: The effect of a 6-minute manual muscle massage on the excitability of the spinal reflex pathway was assessed in 20 subjects. H-reflex recordings were obtained from the right soleus muscle, which was the site being massaged. Skin temperature and antagonist activity were monitored. An A-B-A interrupted-time series design was used consisting of two pretreatment, two treatment (massage), and two post-treatment conditions.

Results: H-reflex amplitudes recorded during both massage conditions were significantly reduced in comparison to all other (before and after) conditions. This decrease could not be explained conclusively by changes in skin temperature, nerve conduction velocity, or antagonist recruitment, thus indicating a decrease in spinal reflex excitability attributable to massage.

Sullivan SJ, Williams L, Seaborne DE, et al (1991). Effects of massage on alpha motoneuron excitability. *Physical Therapy* **71:555–560**

Method: The purpose of this study was to investigate the specificity of the effects of massage (petrissage) on spinal motoneuron excitability as measured by changes in the peak-to-peak amplitude of H-reflex recordings. H-reflexes (and M-responses) were recorded from the distal aspects of the right triceps surae muscle of eight men and eight women, aged 20–37 years, with no neuromuscular impairments of the lower extremities. The H-reflexes were recorded during five control and four experimental conditions (20 trials at each condition). The control conditions preceded and followed each experimental condition, providing a measure of the stability of the H-reflex. Each experimental condition consisted of a 4-minute period of massage of the ipsilateral and contralateral triceps surae and hamstring muscle groups.

Results: The mean peak-to-peak amplitude of the H-reflex was found to be stable across the five control conditions. H-reflex amplitudes recorded during the experimental conditions indicate that massage of the ipsilateral triceps surae resulted in a reduction of the H-reflex in comparison with the pre-test control condition and the remaining experimental conditions. Subsequent analyses indicated a specificity of the effects of massage on the muscle group being massaged.

HEADACHE

Foster KA, Liskin J, Cen S, et al (2004). The Trager approach in the treatment of chronic headache: a pilot study. *Alternative Therapies in Health and Medicine* **10:40–46**

Method: Although the traditional treatment of headache has been pharmacological, there have been many attempts to treat headaches with other methods with mixed levels of success.
Objective: To obtain preliminary data on the efficacy of the Trager approach in the treatment of chronic headache.
Design: Small-scale randomized controlled clinical trial.
Setting: University-based clinic.
Patients: Thirty-three volunteers with a self-reported history of chronic headache and with at least one headache per week for at least 6 months received Trager massage.
Interventions: Medication-only control group, both medication and attention control group, and medication and Trager treatment group.
Main outcome measures: Self-reported frequency, duration, and intensity of headache, medication usage and headache quality of life (HQOL) obtained at baseline and after a 6-week treatment period.
Results: Analyses of variance demonstrated significant improvement in HQOL for the Trager and attention control groups, and reduction in medication usage for the Trager group ($p < 0.05$). Participants randomized to Trager demonstrated a significant decrease in the frequency of headaches ($p = 0.045$), improvement in HQOL ($p = 0.045$), and a 44% decrease in medication usage ($p = 0.03$). Participants randomized to the attention control group demonstrated a significant improvement in HQOL ($p = 0.035$) and a 19% decrease in medication usage ($p = 0.15$). Participants randomized to the no-treatment control group revealed a significant increase in headache duration ($p = 0.025$) and intensity ($p = 0.025$), and a declination in HQOL ($p = 0.035$).
Conclusions: The Trager approach decreased headache frequency and medication usage. Trager and physician attention improved HQOL. A larger, multi-site study is recommended.

Hernandez-Reif M, Field T, Dieter J, et al (1998). Migraine headaches are reduced by massage therapy. *International Journal of Neuroscience* **96:1–11**

Method: Twenty-six adults with migraine headaches were randomly assigned to a massage therapy group, which received twice-weekly 30-minute massages for 5 consecutive weeks, or a wait-list control group.

Results: The massage group reported fewer distress symptoms, less pain, more headache-free days, fewer sleep disturbances and taking fewer analgesics. They also showed increased serotonin levels.

Quinn C, Chandler C, Moraska A (2002). Massage therapy and frequency of chronic tension headaches. *American Journal of Public Health* **92:1657–1661**

Method: This study examined the effects of massage therapy on chronic, non-migraine headache. Four chronic tension headache sufferers (aged 18–55 years) received structured massage therapy treatment directed toward the neck and shoulder muscles during a 4-week period. Data included headache frequency, duration, and intensity prior to and during the treatment period.

Results: Massage therapy was effective in reducing the number of weekly headaches. Headache frequency was significantly reduced within the initial week of massage treatment, and continued for the remainder of the study. A trend toward reduction in average duration of each headache event between the baseline period and the treatment period was also observed. Headache intensity was unaffected by massage treatment.

HIV

Diego MA, Hernandez-Reif M, Field T, et al (2001). HIV adolescents show improved immune function following massage therapy. *International Journal of Neuroscience* **106:35–45**

Method: HIV+ adolescents recruited from a large urban university hospital's outpatient clinic were randomly assigned to receive massage therapy (n = 12) or progressive muscle relaxation (n = 12) two times per week for 12 weeks. To assess treatment effects, participants were assessed for depression, anxiety and immune changes before and after the 12-week treatment period.

Results: Adolescents who received massage therapy versus those who experienced relaxation therapy reported feeling less anxious and they were less depressed and showed enhanced immune function by the end of the 12-week study. Immune changes for the massage therapy group included increased natural killer cell number and the HIV disease progression markers (CD4/CD8 ratio and CD4 number).

Ironson G, Field T, Scafidi F, et al (1996). Massage therapy is associated with enhancement of the immune system's cytotoxic capacity. *International Journal of Neuroscience* **84:205–217**

Method: Twenty-nine gay men (20 HIV+, 9 HIV–) received daily massages for 1 month. A subset of 11 of the HIV+ subjects served as a within-subjects control group (1 month with and without massages).

Results: Major immune findings for the effects of the month of massage included a significant increase in natural killer cell number, natural killer cell activity, and CD8. No changes occurred in HIV disease progression markers. Neuroendocrine findings measured via 24-hour urine samples included a decrease in cortisol and trends toward decreased catecholamines. Decreased anxiety and increased relaxation were significantly correlated with increased NK cell number.

Scafidi F, Field T (1996). Massage therapy improves behavior in neonates born to HIV positive mothers. *Journal of Pediatric Psychology* **21:889–898**

Method: Neonates born to HIV-positive mothers were randomly assigned to a massage therapy or control group. The treatment infants were given three 15-minute massages daily for 10 days.
Results: The massaged group showed superior performance on almost every Brazelton newborn cluster score and had a greater daily weight gain at the end of the treatment period unlike the control group who showed declining performance.

HOSPICE

Meek SS (1993). Effects of slow stroke back massage on relaxation in hospice clients. *Journal of Nursing Scholarship* **25:17–21**

Method: Slow stroke back massage was provided for 30 hospice patients.
Results: The massage was associated with decreases in systolic BP, diastolic BP, and heart rate and an increase in skin temperature.

HOSPITALIZED PATIENTS

Smith MC, Stallings MA, Mariner S, et al (1999). Benefits of massage therapy for hospitalized patients: a descriptive and qualititative evaluation. *Alternative Therapies in Health & Medicine* **5:64–71**

Method: The objective of this study was to assess outcomes of a therapeutic massage program within an acute care setting. One hundred and thirteen patients received one to four massages during the course of their hospital stay.
Results: The most frequently identified outcomes were increased relaxation (98%), a sense of well-being (93%), and positive mood change (88%). More than two-thirds of patients attributed enhanced mobility, greater energy, increased participation in treatment, and faster recovery to massage therapy. 35% stated that benefits lasted more than 1 day.

HYPERTENSION

Hernandez-Reif M, Field T, Krasnegor J, et al (2000). High blood pressure and associated symptoms were reduced by massage therapy. *Journal of Bodywork and Movement Therapies* **4:31–38**

Method: High blood pressure is associated with elevated anxiety, stress and stress hormones, hostility, depression and catecholamines. Massage therapy and progressive muscle relaxation were evaluated as treatments for reducing blood pressure and associated symptoms. Adults who had been diagnosed as hypertensive received ten 30-minute massage sessions over 5 weeks or they were given progressive muscle relaxation instructions (control group).

Results: Sitting diastolic blood pressure decreased after the first and last massage therapy sessions and reclining diastolic blood pressure decreased from the first to the last day of the study. Although both groups reported less anxiety, only the massage therapy group reported less depression and hostility and showed decreased urinary and salivary hormone levels (cortisol). Massage therapy may be effective in reducing diastolic blood pressure and symptoms associated with hypertension.

IMMUNOLOGY

Zeitlin D, Keller SE, Shiflett SC, et al (2000). Immunological effects of massage therapy during acute academic stress. *Psychosomatic Medicine* **62:83–84**

Method: This study examined the immunological effects of massage therapy as a stress-reduction intervention in nine healthy female medical students (aged 21–25 yars). Subjects received a 1-hour full body massage 1 day before an anxiety-provoking academic examination. Blood samples, self-report data (the State component of the State-Trait Anxiety Inventory and a visual analogue scale of perceived stress), and vital signs (respiratory rate, BP, pulse, and temperature) were obtained immediately prior to and after the message. Cell phenotypes of the major cells of the immune system, natural killer cell activity (NKCA), and mitogen-induced lymphocyte stimulation were assessed by standard techniques.

Results: A significant decrease in respiratory rate occurred from pre- to post-massage. Mean anxiety scores decreased from 53 to 27 and mean scores on the visual analogue scale decreased from 76 to 35 from pre- to post-massage. No significant pre- to post-massage lymphocyte responses to mitogens were found, but a significant increase in NKCA occurred post-massage. NKCA correlated negatively with both perceived stress and anxiety. Results suggest that massage reduces subjective and somatic signs of anxiety and that massage may have health benefits beyond and unrelated to its stress-reduction potential.

INFANTS

Agarwal KN, Gupta A, Pushkarna R, et al (2000). Effects of massage and use of oil on growth, blood flow and sleep pattern in infants. *Indian Journal of Medical Research* **112:212–217**

Method: The present study was undertaken to investigate if massage with oils commonly used in the community for massage in infancy is beneficial.

Full-term born healthy infants (n = 125), 6 +/− 1 week of age, weight >3000 g were randomly divided into five groups. Infants received (i) herbal oil, (ii) sesame oil, (iii) mustard oil, or (iv) mineral oil for massage daily for 4 weeks. The fifth group did not receive massage and served as control. The study tools were anthropometric measurements; microhematrocrit; serum proteins, creatinine and creatine phosphokinase; blood flow using colour Doppler and sleep pattern.

Results: Massage improved the weight, length, and midarm and midleg circumferences as compared to infants without massage. However, in the group with sesame oil massage increase in length, midarm and midleg circumferences by 1.0, 0.9 and 0.7 cm, respectively was significant ($p < 0.05$, < 0.01 and < 0.05). There was no change in microhematocrit, serum proteins, albumin, creatinine and creatine phosphokinase between both the groups. The femoral artery blood velocity, diameter and flow improved significantly by 12.6 cm/second, 0.6 cm and 3.55 cm^3/second respectively in the group with sesame oil massage as compared to the control group. Massage improved the post-massage sleep, the maximum being 1.62 hours in the sesame oil group ($p < 0.0001$).

Interpretation & Conclusions: Massage in infancy improves growth and post-massage sleep. However, only sesame oil showed significant benefit.

Cullen C, Field T, Escalona A, et al (2000). Father–infant interactions are enhanced by massage therapy. *Early Child Development and Care* **164:41–47**

Method: Fathers gave their infants daily massages 15 minutes prior to bedtime for 1 month.
Results: By the end of the study, the fathers who massaged their infants were more expressive and showed more enjoyment and more warmth during floor-play interactions with their infants.

Ferber SG, Laudon M, Kuint J, et al (2002). Massage therapy by mothers enhances the adjustment of circadian rhythms to the nocturnal period in full-term infants. *Journal of Developmental and Behavioral Pediatrics* **23:410–415**

Method: This study investigated the effect of massage therapy on phase adjustment of rest-activity and melatonin secretion rhythms to the nocturnal period in full-term infants. Rest-activity of infants was measured by actigraphy before and after 14 days of massage therapy (starting at approximately age 10 days) and subsequently at 6 and 8 weeks of age. 6-Sulphatoxymelatonin (6-SM) was assessed in urine samples at 6, 8, and 12 weeks of age.
Results: At 8 weeks the controls revealed one peak of activity at approximately 12 midnight and another one at approximately 12 noon, whereas in the treated group, a major peak was early in the morning and a secondary peak in the late afternoon. At 12 weeks, nocturnal 6-SM excretions were significantly higher in the treated infants. Thus, massage therapy by mothers in

the perinatal period serves as a strong time cue, enhancing coordination of the developing circadian system with environmental cues.

Field T (1995). Massage therapy for infants and children. [Review]. *Journal of Developmental & Behavioral Pediatrics* **16:105–111**

Data are reviewed on the effects of massage therapy on infants and children with various medical conditions. The infants include: premature infants, cocaine-exposed infants, HIV-exposed infants, infants parented by depressed mothers, and full-term infants without medical problems. The childhood conditions include: abuse (sexual and physical), asthma, autism, burns, cancer, developmental delays, dermatitis, diabetes, eating disorders (anorexia and bulimia), juvenile rheumatoid arthritis, post-traumatic stress disorder, and psychiatric problems. Generally, the massage therapy has resulted in lower anxiety and stress hormones and improved clinical course. Having grandparent volunteers and parents give the therapy enhances their own wellness and provides a cost-effective treatment for the children.

Field T (2001). Massage therapy facilitates weight gain in preterm infants. *Current Directions in Psychological Science* **10:51–54**

Method: Studies from several labs have documented a 31–47% greater weight gain in preterm newborns receiving massage therapy (three 15-minute sessions for 5–10 days) compared with standard medical treatment. Although the underlying mechanism for this relationship between massage therapy and weight gain has not yet been established, possibilities that have been explored in studies with both humans and rats include (1) increased protein synthesis, (2) increased vagal activity that releases food-absorption hormones like insulin and enhances gastric motility, and (3) decreased cortisol levels leading to increased oxytocin. In addition, functional magnetic resonance imaging studies are being conducted to assess the effects of touch therapy on brain development.

Field T, Hernandez-Reif M (2001). Sleep problems in infants decrease following massage therapy. *Early Child Development and Care* **168:95–104**

Method: Infants and toddlers (mean age = 1.5 years) with sleep onset problems were given daily massages by their parents for 15 minutes prior to bedtime for 1 month.
Results: Based on parent diaries the massaged versus the control children (who were read bedtime stories) showed fewer sleep delay behaviors and had a shorter latency to sleep onset by the end of the study. Forty-five minute behavior observations by an independent observer also revealed more time awake, alert and active and more positive affect in the massaged children by the end of the study.

Field T, Grizzle N, Scafidi F, et al (1996). Massage therapy for infants of depressed mothers. *Infant Behavior and Development* **19:109–114**

Method: Forty full-term 1- to 3-month-old infants born to depressed adolescent mothers who were low socieconomic status (SES) and single parents were given 15 minutes of either massage or rocking for 2 days per week for a 6-week period.

Results: The infants who experienced massage therapy compared to infants in the rocking control group spent more time in active alert and active awake states, cried less, and had lower salivary cortisol levels, suggesting lower stress. After the massage versus the rocking sessions, the infants spent less time in an active awake state, suggesting that massage may be more effective than rocking for inducing sleep. Over the 6-week period, the massage-therapy infants gained more weight, showed greater improvement on emotionality, sociability, and soothability temperament dimensions and had greater decreases in urinary stress catecholamines/hormones (norepinephrine, epinephrine, cortisol).

Huhtala V, Lehtonen L, Heinonen R, et al (2000). Infant massage compared with crib vibrator in the treatment of colicky infants. *Pediatrics* **105:E84**

Method: To evaluate the effectiveness of infant massage compared with that of a crib vibrator in the treatment of infantile colic. Infants <7 weeks of age and perceived as colicky by their parents were randomly assigned to an infant massage group (n = 28) or a crib vibrator group (n = 30). Three daily intervention periods were recommended in both groups. Parents recorded infant crying and given interventions in a structured cry diary that was kept for 1 week before (baseline) and for 3 weeks during the intervention. Parents were interviewed after the first and third weeks of intervention to obtain their evaluation of the effectiveness of the given massage or crib vibration.

Results: At baseline, the mean amount of total crying was 3.6 (standard deviation: 1.4) hours/day in the massage group infants and 4.2 (2.0) hours/day in the vibrator group infants. The mean amount of colicky crying was 2.1 (standard deviation: 1.1) hours/day and 2.9 (1.5) hours/day, respectively. The mean number of daily intervention periods was 2.2 in both groups. Over the 4-week study, the amount of total and colicky crying decreased significantly in both intervention groups. The reduction in crying was similar in the study groups: total crying decreased by a mean 48% in the massage group and by 47% in the vibrator group, and colicky crying decreased by 64% and 52%, respectively. The amount of other crying (total crying minus colicky crying) remained stable in both groups over the intervention. 93% of the parents in both groups reported that colic symptoms decreased over the 3-week intervention, and 61% of the parents in the massage group and 63% of the parents in the crib vibrator group perceived the 3-week intervention as colic-reducing.

Conclusions: Infant massage was comparable to the use of a crib vibrator in reducing crying in colicky infants. We suggest that the decrease of total and colicky crying in the present study reflects more the natural course of early infant crying and colic than a specific effect of the interventions.

Scafidi F, Field T (1996). Massage therapy improves behavior in neonates born to HIV-positive mothers. *Journal of Pediatric Psychology* **21:889–897**

Method: 28 neonates born to HIV-positive mothers were randomly assigned to a massage therapy or control group. The treatment infants were given three 15-minute massages daily for 10 days.

Results: The massaged group showed superior performance on almost every Brazelton newborn cluster score and had a greater daily weight gain at the end of the treatment period, unlike the control group who showed declining performance.

Scholtz K, Samuels CA (1992). Neonatal bathing and massage intervention with fathers: behavioral effects 12 weeks after birth of the first baby. *International Journal of Behavioral Development* **15:67–81**

Method: Australian families with first-born babies were studied for effects of a 4-week-postpartum training program (demonstration of baby massage and the Burleigh Relaxation Bath technique), with emphasis on the father–infant relationship. Sixteen families were assigned to the treatment group and 16 served as controls.

Results: At the 12-week home observation, the treatment group infants greeted their fathers with more eye contact, smiling, vocalizing, reaching, and orienting responses and showed less avoidance behaviors. During a 10-minute observation, the treatment group fathers showed greater involvement with their infants.

Uvnas-Moberg K, Widstrom AM, Marchini G, et al (1987). Release of GI hormones in mother and infant by sensory stimulation. [Review]. *Acta Paediatrica Scandinavia* **76:851–860**

Sensory stimulation is of great importance for the growth and the physiological and psychological development of infants. Supplementary sensory stimulation such as non-nutritive sucking and tactile stimulation has been shown to increase the growth rate and the maturation of premature infants. In human neonates non-nutritive sucking has a vagally-mediated influence on the levels of some gastrointestinal hormones. In animal experiments afferent electrical stimulation of the sciatic nerve at low intensity leads to an activation of the vagal nerve and to a consequent release of vagally-controlled gastrointestinal hormones such as gastrin and cholecystokinin. We therefore assume that both non-nutritive sucking and tactile stimulation trigger the activity of sensory nerves which leads to a release of vagally regulated gut hormones. Since gut hormones stimulate gastrointestinal motor and secretory activity and the growth of the gastrointestinal tract, and enhance the glucose-induced insulin release, they may contribute to the beneficial effects on maturation and growth caused by sensory stimulation. In the breast-feeding situation, the sucking of the child elicits similar reflexes in the mother leading to an activation of the maternal gut endocrine system and a consequent increase in energy uptake.

JOB STRESS

Cady SH, Jones GE (1997). Massage therapy as a workplace intervention for reduction of stress. *Perceptual & Motor Skills* 84:157–158

Method: The effectiveness of a 15-minute, on-site massage while seated in a chair was evaluated for reducing stress as indicated by blood pressure. Fifty-two employed participants' blood pressures were measured before and after a 15-minute massage at work.

Results: Analyses showed a significant reduction in participants' systolic and diastolic blood pressure after receiving the massage.

Field T, Ironson G, Scafidi F, et al (1996). Massage therapy reduces anxiety and enhances EEG pattern of alertness and math computations. *International Journal of Neuroscience* 86:197–205

Method: Twenty-six adults were given a chair massage and 24 control group adults were asked to relax in the massage chair for 15 minutes, two times per week for 5 weeks. On the first and last days of the study they were monitored for EEG before, during and after the sessions. In addition, before and after the sessions they performed math computations, they completed POMS Depression and State Anxiety Scales and they provided a saliva sample for cortisol. At the beginning of the sessions they completed Life Events, Job Stress and POMS Depression Scales.

Results: Analyses revealed the following: (1) frontal delta power increased for both groups, suggesting relaxation; (2) the massage group showed decreased frontal alpha and beta power (suggesting enhanced alertness); (3) the massage group showed increased speed and accuracy on math computations; (4) anxiety levels were lower following the massage and mood state was less depressed following both the massage and control sessions; (5) salivary cortisol levels were lower following the massage; and (6) at the end of the 5-week period depression scores were lower for both groups, but the job stress score was lower only for the massage group.

Field T, Quintino O, Henteleff T, et al (1997). Job stress reduction therapies. *Alternative Therapies in Health and Medicine* 3:54–56

Method: The immediate effects of brief massage therapy, music relaxation with visual imagery, muscle relaxation, and social support group sessions were assessed in 100 hospital employees at a major public hospital.

Results: Each of the groups reported decreases in anxiety, depression, fatigue, and confusion, as well as increased vigor following the sessions.

JUVENILE RHEUMATOID ARTHRITIS

Field T, Hernandez-Reif M, Seligman S, et al (1997). Juvenile rheumatoid arthritis: benefits from massage therapy. *Journal of Pediatric Psychology* 22:607–617

Method: In this study, children with mild to moderate juvenile rheumatoid arthritis were massaged by their parents 15 minutes a day for 30 days (and a control group engaged in relaxation therapy).

Results: The children's anxiety and stress hormone (cortisol) levels were immediately decreased by the massage, and over the 30-day period their pain decreased on self-reports, parent reports, and their physician's assessment of pain (both the incidence and severity) and pain-limiting activities.

LABOR PAIN

Chang MY, Wang SY, Chen CH (2002). Effects of massage on pain and anxiety during labour: a randomized controlled trial in Taiwan. *Journal of Advanced Nursing* **38:68–73**

Method: To investigate the effects of massage on pain reaction and anxiety during labor. Labor pain is a challenging issue for nurses designing intervention protocols. Massage is an ancient technique that has been widely employed during labor; however, relatively little study has been undertaken examining the effects of massage on women in labor. A randomized controlled study was conducted between September 1999 and January 2000. Sixty primiparous women expected to have a normal childbirth at a regional hospital in southern Taiwan were randomly assigned to either the experimental (n = 30) or the control (n = 30) group. The experimental group received massage intervention whereas the control group did not. The nurse-rated present behavioral intensity (PBI) was used as a measure of labor pain. Anxiety was measured with the visual analog scale for anxiety (VASA). The intensity of pain and anxiety between the two groups was compared in the latent phase (cervix dilated 3–4 cm), active phase (5–7 cm) and transitional phase (8–10 cm).

Results: In both groups, there was a relatively steady increase in pain intensity and anxiety level as labor progressed. A t-test demonstrated that the experimental group had significantly lower pain reactions in the latent, active and transitional phases. Anxiety levels were only significantly different between the two groups in the latent phase. Twenty-six of the 30 (87%) experimental group subjects reported that massage was helpful, providing pain relief and psychological support during labour.

Conclusions: Findings suggest that massage is a cost-effective nursing intervention that can decrease pain and anxiety during labour, and partners' participation in massage can positively influence the quality of women's birth experiences.

Chung UL, Hung LC, Kuo SC, et al (2003). Effects of LI4 and BL67 acupressure on labor pain and uterine contractions in the first stage of labor. *Journal of Nursing Research* **11:251–260**

Method: Acupressure is said to promote the circulation of blood and qi, the harmony of yin and yang, and the secretion of neurotransmitters, thus maintaining the normal functions of the human body and providing comfort. However, there has been little research-based evidence to support the positive effects of acupressure in the area of obstetric nursing. The purpose of this study is to determine the effect of LI4 and BL67 acupressure on labor pain and uterine contractions during the first stage of labor. An experimental study with a pre-test and post-test control group design was utilized. A total of 127 parturient women were randomly assigned to three groups. Each group received only one of the following treatments, LI4 and BL67 acupressure, light skin stroking, or no treatment/conversation only. Data collected from the VAS and external fetal monitoring strips were used for analysis.

Results: A significant difference in decreased labor pain during the active phase of the first stage of labor among the three groups. There was no significant difference in effectiveness of uterine contractions during the first stage of labor among the three groups. Results of the study confirmed the effect of LI4 and BL67 acupressure in lessening labor pain during the active phase of the first stage of labor. There were no verified effects on uterine contractions.

Field T, Hernandez-Reif M, Taylor S, et al (1997). Labor pain is reduced by massage therapy. *Journal of Psychosomatic Obstetrics and Gynecology* **18:286–291**

Method: Twenty-eight women were recruited from prenatal classes and randomly assigned to receive massage in addition to coaching in breathing from their partners during labor, or to receive coaching in breathing alone (a technique learned during prenatal classes).

Results: The massaged mothers reported a decrease in depressed mood and anxiety and more positive affect following the first massage during labor. In addition, the massaged mothers had significantly shorter labor, a shorter hospital stay and less postpartum depression.

LEARNING—see cognition

LEUKEMIA

Field T, Cullen C, Diego M, et al (2001). Leukemia immune changes following massage therapy. *Journal of Bodywork and Movement Therapies* **5:271–274**

Method: Twenty children with leukemia were provided with daily massage therapy by their parents and were compared to a standard treatment control group.

Results: Following a month of massage therapy, depressed mood decreased in the children's parents, and the children's white blood cell and neutrophil counts increased.

LOWER BACK PAIN

Cherkin DC, Eisenberg D, Sherman KJ, et al (2001). Randomized trial comparing traditional Chinese medical acupuncture, therapeutic massage, and self-care education for chronic low back pain. *Archives of Internal Medicine* **161:1081–1088**

Method: 262 patients who had persistent back pain received traditional Chinese medical acupuncture, therapeutic massage, or self-care educational materials for up to 10 massage or acupuncture visits over 10 weeks.

Results: At 10 weeks, massage was superior to self-care on the symptom scale and the disability scale. Massage was also superior to acupuncture on the disability scale. The massage group used the least medications and had the lowest costs of subsequent care.

Degan M, Fabris F, Vanin F, et al (2000). The effectiveness of foot reflexotherapy on chronic pain associated with a herniated disk. *[Italian] Professioni Infermieristiche* **53:80–87**

Method: A group of 40 persons suffering almost exclusively from a lumbar-sacral disc hernia received three treatments of reflexology massage for a week.

Results: 25 persons (62.5%) reported a reduction in pain, (rating at 0.75 on a scale of 0–4).

Ernst E (1999). Massage therapy for low back pain: a systematic review [In Process Citation]. *Journal of Pain Symptom Management* **17:65–69**

Massage therapy is frequently employed for low back pain. The aim of this sytematic review was to find the evidence for or against its efficacy in this indication. Four random clinical trials were located in which massage was tested as a monotherapy for low back pain. All were burdened with major methodological flaws. One of these studies suggests that massage is superior to no treatment. Two trials imply that it is equally effective as spinal manipulation or transcutaneous electrical stimulation. One study suggests that it is less effective than spinal manipulation. It is concluded that too few trials of massage therapy exist for a reliable evaluation of its efficacy. Massage seems to have some potential as a therapy for low back pain.

Furlan AD, Brosseau L, Imamura M, et al (2000). Massage for low back pain. *Cochrane Database of Systematic Reviews* **2:CD001929**

Method: This study assessed the effects of massage therapy for non-specific low back pain. Two reviewers blinded to authors, journal and institutions selected the studies, assessed the methodological quality using the criteria recommended by the Cochrane Back Review Group, and extracted the data using standardized forms. The studies were analyzed in a qualitative way due to heterogeneity of population, massage technique, comparison groups, timing and type of outcome measured.

Results: Nine publications reporting on eight randomized trials were included. Three had low and five had high methodological quality scores. One study was published in German and the rest in English. Massage was compared to an inert treatment (sham laser) in one study that showed that massage was superior, especially if given in combination with exercises and education. In the other seven studies, massage was compared to different active treatments. They showed that massage was inferior to manipulation and TENS; massage was equal to corsets and exercises; and massage was superior to relaxation therapy, acupuncture and self-care education. The beneficial effects of massage in patients with chronic low back pain lasted at least 1 year after the end of the treatment. One study comparing two different techniques of massage concluded in favour of acupuncture massage over classic (Swedish) massage.

Hernandez-Reif M, Field T, Krasnegor J, et al (2001). Lower back pain is reduced and range of motion increased after massage therapy. *International Journal of Neuroscience* **106:131–145**

Method: Twenty-four adults (12 women) with lower back pain were randomly assigned to a massage therapy or a progressive muscle relaxation group. Sessions were 30 minutes long, twice a week for 5 weeks. On the first and last days of the 5-week study participants completed questionnaires, provided a urine sample and were assessed for range of motion.

Results: By the end of the study, the massage therapy group, as compared to the relaxation group, reported experiencing less pain, depression, anxiety and improved sleep. They also showed improved trunk flexion, and their serotonin and dopamine levels were higher.

Hsieh LL, Kuo CH, Yen MF, et al (2004). A randomized controlled clinical trial for low back pain treated by acupressure and physical therapy. *Preventative Medicine* **39:168–176**

Method: Although acupressure has been reported to be effective in managing various types of pain, its efficacy in relieving pain associated with low back pain (LBP) remains unclear. The aim of this study is to compare the efficacy of acupressure with that of physical therapy in reducing low back pain. A randomized controlled clinical trial in an orthopedic referral hospital in Taiwan was conducted between December 20, 2000, and March 2, 2001. A total of 146 participants with chronic low back pain were randomly assigned to the acupressure group (69) or the physical therapy group (77), each with a different treatment technique. Self-appraised pain scores were obtained before treatment as baseline and after treatment as outcomes using the Chinese version of Short-Form Pain Questionnaire (SF-PQ).

Results: There were no significant differences in baseline characteristics among patients randomized into the two groups. The mean of post-treatment pain score after a 4-week treatment (2.28, SD = 2.62) in the acupressure group was significantly lower than that in the physical therapy group (5.05, SD = 5.11) (p = 0.0002). At the 6-month follow-up assessment, the mean of pain score in the acupressure group (1.08, SD = 1.43) was still significantly lower than that in the physical therapy group(3.15, SD = 3.62) (p = 0.0004).

Conclusions: Our results suggest that acupressure is another effective alternative medicine in reducing low back pain, although the standard operating procedures involved with acupressure treatment should be carefully assessed in the future.

Kalauokalani D, Cherkin DC, Sherman KJ, et al (2001). Lessons from a trial of acupuncture and massage for low back pain: patient expectations and treatment effects. *Spine* **26:1418–1424**

Method: 135 patients with chronic low back pain who received acupuncture or massage were studied. Study participants were asked to describe their expectations regarding the helpfulness of each treatment on a scale of 0–10. The primary outcome was level of function at 10 weeks as measured by the modified Roland Disability scale.

Results: Improved function was observed for 86% of the participants with higher expectations for the treatment they received, as compared with 68% of those with lower expectations. Patients who expected greater benefit from massage than from acupuncture were more likely to experience better outcomes with massage than with acupuncture, and vice versa.

Kolich M, Taboun SM, Mohamed AI (2000). Low back muscle activity in an automobile seat with a lumbar massage system. *International Journal of Occupational Safety & Ergonomics* **6:113–128**

Method: This investigation was conducted to determine the effects of a massaging lumbar support system on low back muscle activity. The apparatus was a luxury-level automobile seat massage. The dependent variable was the change in the EMG signal.

Results: 1 minute of lumbar massage every 5 minutes was found to have a beneficial effect on low back muscle activity (as compared to no massage).

Pope MH, Phillips RB, Haugh LD, et al (1994). A prospective randomized three-week trial of spinal manipulation, transcutaneous muscle stimulation, massage and corset in the treatment of subacute low back pain. *Spine* **19:2571–2577**

Method: A randomized prospective trial of manipulation, massage, corset and transcutaneous muscle stimulation (TMS) was conducted in patients with subacute low back pain. The authors determined the relative efficacy of chiropractic treatment to massage, corset, and TMS. Patients were enrolled for a period of 3 weeks. They were evaluated once a week by questionnaires, visual analog scale, range of motion, maximum voluntary extension effort, straight leg raising and Biering-Sorensen fatigue test.

Results: After 3 weeks, the manipulation group scored the greatest improvements in flexion and pain while the massage group had the best extension effort and fatigue time, and the muscle stimulation group the best extension.

Preyde M (2000). Effectiveness of massage therapy for subacute low-back pain: a randomized controlled trial. *Canadian Medical Association Journal* **162:1815–1820**

Method: The effectiveness of massage therapy for low-back pain has not been documented. This randomized controlled trial compared comprehensive massage therapy (soft-tissue manipulation, remedial exercise and posture education), two components of massage therapy and placebo in the treatment of subacute (between 1 week and 8 months) low-back pain. Subjects with subacute low-back pain were randomly assigned to one of four groups: comprehensive massage therapy (n = 25), soft-tissue manipulation only (n = 25), remedial exercise with posture education only (n = 22) or a placebo of sham laser therapy (n = 26). Each subject received six treatments within approximately 1 month. Outcome measures obtained at baseline, after treatment and at 1-month follow-up consisted of the Roland Disability Questionnaire (RDQ), the McGill Pain Questionnaire (PPI and PRI), the State Anxiety Index and the Modified Schober test (lumbar range of motion).
Results: Of the 107 subjects who passed screening, 98 (92%) completed post-treatment tests and 91 (85%) completed follow-up tests. Statistically significant differences were noted after treatment and at follow-up. The comprehensive massage therapy group had improved function (mean RDQ score 1.54 vs 2.86–6.5, $p < 0.001$), less intense pain (mean PPI score 0.42 vs 1.18–1.75, $p < 0.001$) and a decrease in the quality of pain (mean PRI score 2.29 vs 4.55–7.71, $p = 0.006$) compared with the other three groups. Clinical significance was evident for the comprehensive massage therapy group and the soft-tissue manipulation group on the measure of function. At 1-month follow-up 63% of subjects in the comprehensive massage therapy group reported no pain as compared with 27% of the soft-tissue manipulation group, 14% of the remedial exercise group and 0% of the sham laser therapy group.
Interpretation: Patients with subacute low-back pain were shown to benefit from massage therapy, as regulated by the College of Massage Therapists of Ontario and delivered by experienced massage therapists.

Yip YB, Tse SH (2004). The effectiveness of relaxation acupoint stimulation and acupressure with aromatic lavender essential oil for non-specific low back pain in Hong Kong: a randomized controlled trial. *Complementary Therapies in Medicine* **12:28–37**

Method: This study assessed the effect of acupoint stimulation with electrodes combined with acupressure using an aromatic essential oil (lavender) as an add-on-treatment on pain relief and enhancing the physical functional activities among adults with subacute or chronic non-specific low back pain.

The intervention was an eight-session relaxation acupoint stimulation followed by acupressure with lavender oil over a 3-week period. The control group received usual care only.

Results: One week after the end of treatment, the intervention group had 39% greater reduction in VAS pain intensity than the control group, improved walking time and greater lateral spine flexion range.

LYMPHATICS

Eliska O, Eliskova M (1995) Are peripheral lymphatics damaged by high pressure manual massage? *Lymphology* 28:21–30

Method: Massage of the foot in men and the hindpaw in dogs was performed by applying external pressures of 70–100 mmHg for a period of 1, 3, 5, and 10 minutes with a frequency of 25 strokes per minute. This protocol was performed on individuals without edema, on dogs with experimental lymphedema and men with post-thrombotic venous edema.

Results: After 10 minutes of forceful massage, focal damage of lymphatics was present. In a group of dogs with lymphedema and men with post-thrombotic venous edema, the alteration of lymphatics was greater than in normal individuals and evident only after 3–5 minutes of massage. At first, the forceful massage affected the endothelial lining of the initial lymphatics. Alterations of lymphatic collectors were visible later. The fluid in lymphedema was translocated by massage using high pressure from the interstitium into the lumen of lymphatics by means of the open junctions and by artificial cracks that develop from injury to the lymphatic wall. Vigorous massage in lymphedema also produces loosening of subcutaneous connective tissue, formation of large tissue channels and release of lipid droplets that enter the lymphatics. By this mechanism, massage helps reduce the amount of fat cells in the lymphedematous leg.

MOTONEURON

Sullivan SJ, Williams L, Seaborne DE, et al (1991). Effects of massage on alpha motoneuron excitability. *Physical Therapy* 71:555–560

Method: The purpose of this study was to investigate the specificity of the effects of massage (petrissage) on spinal motoneuron excitability as measured by changes in the peak-to-peak amplitude of H-reflex recordings. H-reflexes (and M-responses) were recorded from the distal aspects of the right triceps surae muscle of eight men and eight women, aged 20–37 years, with no neuromuscular impairments of the lower extremities. The H-reflexes were recorded during five control and four experimental conditions (20 trials at each condition). The control conditions (C1–C5) preceded and followed each experimental condition, providing a measure of the stability of the H-reflex. Each experimental condition consisted of a 4-minute period of massage of the ipsilateral and contralateral triceps surae and hamstring muscle groups (ITS, CTS, IHS, and CHS, respectively).

Results: The mean peak-to-peak amplitude of the H-reflex was found to be stable (range = 1.91–1.95 mV) across the five control conditions. H-reflex amplitudes recorded during the experimental conditions indicate that massage of the ITS resulted in a reduction of the H-reflex (0.83 mV) in comparison with the pre-test control condition (C1) and the remaining experimental conditions (range = 1.77–2.23 mV) This difference was significant, and subsequent Newman–Keuls tests indicated a specificity of the effects of massage on the muscle group being massaged.

MULTIPLE SCLEROSIS

Hernandez-Reif M, Field T, Theakston H (1998). Multiple sclerosis patients benefit from massage therapy. *Journal of Bodywork and Movement Therapies* **2:168–174**

Method: Twenty-four adults with multiple sclerosis were randomly assigned to a standard medical treatment control group or a massage therapy group that received 45-minute massages twice a week for 5 weeks.

Results: The massage group had lower anxiety and less depressed mood immediately following the massage sessions and by the end of the study they had improved self-esteem, better body image and image of disease progression, and enhanced social functioning.

Siev-Ner I, Gamus D, Lerner-Geva L, et al (2003). Reflexology treatment relieves symptoms of multiple sclerosis: a randomized controlled study. *Multiple Sclerosis* **9:356–361**

Method: To evaluate the effect of reflexology on symptoms of multiple sclerosis (MS) in a randomized, sham-controlled clinical trial. Seventy-one MS patients were randomized to either study or control group, to receive an 11-week treatment. Reflexology treatment included manual pressure on specific points in the feet and massage of the calf area. The control group received nonspecific massage of the calf area. The intensity of paresthesias, urinary symptoms, muscle strength and spasticity was assessed in a masked fashion at the beginning of the study, after 1.5 months of treatment, end of study and at 3 months of follow-up.

Results: Fifty-three patients completed this study. Significant improvement in the differences in mean scores of paresthesias ($p = 0.01$), urinary symptoms ($p = 0.03$) and spasticity ($p = 0.03$) was detected in the reflexology group. Improvement with borderline significance was observed in the differences in mean scores of muscle strength between the reflexology group and the controls ($p = 0.06$). The improvement in the intensity of paresthesias remained significant at three months of follow-up ($p = 0.04$).

Conclusions: Specific reflexology treatment was of benefit in alleviating motor; sensory and urinary symptoms in MS patients.

NAUSEA

Ming JL, Kuo BI, Lin JG, et al (2002). The efficacy of acupressure to prevent nausea and vomiting in post-operative patients. *Journal of Advanced Nursing* 39:343–351

Method: Post-operative nausea and vomiting is a common complication following general anaesthesia. Traditional Chinese medicine indicates that acupressure therapy may reduce nausea and vomiting in certain ailments. The aim of this study was to examine the effect of stimulating two acupressure points on prevention of post-operative nausea and vomiting. A randomized block experimental design was used. The Rhodes Index of Nausea, Vomiting and Retching (INVR) questionnaire was used as a tool to measure incidence. To control the motion sickness variable, the subjects who underwent functional endoscopic sinus surgery (FESS) under general anaesthesia were randomly assigned to a finger-pressing group, a wrist-band group, and a control group. There were 150 subjects in total with each group consisting of 50 subjects. The acupoints and treatment times were similar in the finger-pressing group and wrist-band pressing group, whereas only conversation was employed in the control group.

Results: Significant differences in the incidence of the post-operative nausea and vomiting were found between the acupressure, wrist-band, and control groups, with a reduction in the incidence rate of nausea from 73.0% to 43.2% and vomiting incidence rate from 90.5% to 42.9% in the former. The amount of vomitus and the degree of discomfort were, respectively, less and lower in the former group.

Conclusion: In view of the total absence of side-effects in acupressure, its application is worthy of use. This study confirmed the effectiveness of acupressure in preventing post-operative nausea and vomiting.

NEWBORN

Kim TI, Shin YH, White-Traut RC (2003). Multisensory intervention improves physical growth and illness rates in Korean orphaned newborn infants. *Research in Nursing & Health* 26:424–433

Method: The purpose of this study was to evaluate the effectiveness of a multisensory intervention on the physical growth and health of Korean orphaned infants. Fifty-eight full-term infants were randomly assigned to a control (n = 28) or an experimental (n = 30) group within 14 days post-birth. In addition to receiving the routine orphanage care, infants in the experimental group received 15 minutes of auditory (female voice), tactile (massage), and visual (eye-to-eye contact) stimulation twice a day, 5 days a week, for 4 weeks.

Results: Compared to the control group, the experimental group had gained significantly more weight and had larger increases in length and head circumference after the 4-week intervention period and at 6 months of age. In addition, the experimental group had significantly fewer illnesses and clinic visits. These data demonstrate that multisensory intervention in conjunction with human/social contact may be effective in facilitating growth for newborn infants placed in orphanages.

OBSTETRICS

Ueda W, Katatoka Y, Sagara Y (1993). Effect of gentle massage on regression of sensory analgesia during epidurals. *Anesthesia & Analgesia* 76:783–785

Method: Epigastric massage was used to assess the regression of the sensory analgesia of the epidural block. Sixteen patients, who underwent minor obstetric or gynecologic surgery under epidural block with lidocaine, were divided into two groups. Group A was the control group and Group B received gentle massage of the epigastric area for 30 minutes.

Results: The regression of sensory analgesia in Group B was significantly faster than in Group A 30 minutes after the massage. The authors concluded that peripheral sensory stimulation as weak as gentle massage may initiate a series of indirect mechanisms that lead to accelerated regression of sensory analgesia.

OIL VS NO OIL

Field T, Schanberg S, Davalos M, et al (1996). Massage with oil has more positive effects on normal infants. *Pre- and Perinatal Psychology Journal* 11:75–80

Method: Sixty 1-month-old normal infants were randomly assigned to a massage group with oil and a massage group without oil. Massage had a soothing/calming influence on the infants, particularly when given with oil.

Results: The infants who received massage with oil were less active, showed fewer stress behaviors and head averting, and their saliva cortisol levels decreased more. In addition, vagal activity increased more following massage with oil versus massage without oil.

OXYTOCIN

Agren C, Lundeberg T, Uvnas-Moberg K, et al (1995). The oxytocin antagonist 1-deamino-2-D-Tyr-(Oet)-4-Thr-8-Orn-oxytocin reverses the increase in the withdrawal response latency to thermal, but not mechanical nociceptive stimuli following oxytocin administration or massage-like stroking in rats. *Neuroscience Letters* 18:49–52

Method: In this study the effect of exogenous oxytocin and of massage-like stroking on the withdrawal latency responses to heat and mechanical nociceptive stimulation were investigated in rats. A hot-plate test was used to assess withdrawal responses.

Results: Exogenous oxytocin and stroking (a low frequency mechanical stimulation) significantly increased the withdrawal latencies in response to mechanical and to thermal nociceptive stimuli. The effect of oxytocin and of stroking on the hot-plate test was reversed by an oxytocin antagonist directed against the uterine receptor. In contrast, the antagonist did not affect the prolonged response latency in the mechanical nociceptive stimulation test following either exogenous oxytocin or stroking. These results support the view that (1) oxytocin administration affects directly nociceptive related behaviour in response to heat stimulation, and (2) massage-like stroking may have an anti-nociceptive effect via activation of oxytocinergic mechanisms. Since the response to mechanical stimulation was not blocked by the antagonist the mechanisms mediating the withdrawal latency to heat and mechanical stimulation could be different.

Kurosawa M, Lundeberg T, Agren G, et al (1995). Massage-like stroking of the abdomen lowers blood pressure in anesthetized rats: influence of oxytocin. *Journal of the Autonomic Nervous System* **56:26–30**

Method: The aim of this study was to determine how massage-like stroking of the abdomen in rats influences arterial blood pressure. The participation of oxytocinergic mechanisms in this effect was also investigated. The ventral and/or lateral sides of the abdomen were stroked at a speed of 20 cm/s with a frequency of 0.017–0.67 Hz in pentobarbital anesthetized, artificially ventilated rats. Arterial blood pressure was recorded with a pressure transducer via a catheter in the carotid artery.

Results: Stroking of the ventral, or both ventral and lateral sides of the abdomen for 1 minute with a frequency of 0.67 Hz caused a marked decrease in arterial blood pressure (approx. 50 mmHg). After cessation of the stimulation blood pressure returned to the control level within 1 minute. The maximum decrease in blood pressure was achieved at frequencies of 0.083 Hz or more. Stroking only the lateral sides of the abdomen elicited a significantly smaller decrease in blood pressure (approx. 30 mmHg decrease) than stroking the ventral side. The decrease in blood pressure caused by stroking was not altered by s.c. administration of an oxytocin antagonist directed against the uterine receptor. In contrast, the administration of 0.1 mg/kg of oxytocin diminished the effect, which was antagonized by a simultaneous injection of the oxytocin antagonist. These results indicate that the massage-like stroking of the abdomen decreases blood pressure in anesthetized rats. This effect does not involve intrinsic oxytocinergic transmission. However, since exogenously applied oxytocin was found to diminish the effect of stroking, oxytocin may exert an inhibitory modulatory effect on this reflex arc.

Matthiesen AS, Ransjo-Arvidson AB, Nissen E, et al (2001). Postpartum maternal oxytocin release by newborns: effects of infant hand massage and sucking. *Birth* **28:13–19**

Method: Hand movements and sucking behavior were studied in healthy term newborns who were placed skin-to-skin on their mothers' chests. Ten vaginally delivered infants whose mothers had not been exposed to maternal analgesia were video-recorded from birth until the first breastfeeding.

Results: Infants used their hands to explore and stimulate their mother's breast in preparation for the first breastfeeding. When the infants were sucking, the massage-like hand movements stopped and started again when the infants made a sucking pause. Periods of increased massage-like hand movements or sucking of the mother's breast were followed by an increase in maternal oxytocin levels.

PAIN

Hasson D, Arnetz B, Jelveus L, et al (2004). A randomized clinical trial of the treatment effects of massage compared to relaxation tape recordings on diffuse long-term pain. *Psychotherapy and Psychosomatics* **73:17–24**

Method: Long-term musculoskeletal pain is a common problem in primary health care settings that is difficult to treat. Two common treatments are mental relaxation and massage. Scientific studies show contradictory results. Furthermore, many studies lack long-term follow-up even though it is a chronic disorder. The purpose of this randomized clinical trial was to assess possible effects of massage as compared to listening to relaxation tapes in conditions of 'diffuse' and long-term musculoskeletal pain. 129 patients from primary health care suffering from long-term musculoskeletal pain were randomized to either a massage or mental relaxation group, and assessed before, during and after treatment.

Results: During treatment there was a significant improvement in the three main outcome measures: self-rated health, mental energy, and muscle pain only in the massage group as compared to the relaxation group. However, at the 3-month post-treatment follow-up, there was a significant worsening in the outcome measures (time × group effect $p < 0.05$) back to initial rating levels in the massage group as compared to no changes in the relaxation group. Massage, but not mental relaxation, is beneficial in attenuating diffuse musculoskeletal symptoms. Beneficial effects were registered only during treatment. This lack of long-term benefits could be due to the short treatment period or treatments such as these do not address the underlying causes of pain. Future studies of long-term pain should include longer treatment periods and post-treatment follow-up. It might also be worthwhile assessing the long-term benefits from booster treatment after the initial intense treatment period.

Katz J, Wowk A, Culp D, et al (1999). Pain and tension are reduced among hospital nurses after on-site massage treatments: a pilot study. *Journal of Perianesthesia Nursing* **14:128–133**

Method: Tension and pain are common occupational hazards of modern-day nursing, especially given recent changes to the health care system. The aims of this pilot study were (1) to evaluate the feasibility of carrying out a series of eight 15-minute workplace-based massage treatments, and (2) to determine whether massage therapy reduced pain and stress experienced by nursing staff at a large teaching hospital. Twelve hospital staff (10 registered nurses and 2 nonmedical ward staff) working in a large tertiary care center volunteered to participate. Participants received up to eight, workplace-based, 15-minute Swedish massage treatments provided by registered massage therapists. Pain, tension, relaxation, and the Profile of Mood States were measured before and after each massage session.

Results: Pain intensity and tension levels were significantly lower after massage. In addition, relaxation levels and overall mood state improved significantly after treatments.

Kubsch SM, Neveau T, Vandertie K (2000). Effect of cutaneous stimulation on pain reduction in emergency department patients. *Complementary Therapies in Nursing & Midwifery* **6:25–32**

Method: Tactile stimulation was used with 50 emergency department patients to relieve pain. Another objective was to determine the effect of tactile stimulation on blood pressure and heart rate.

Results: Following stimulation, subjects reported significantly reduced pain, and demonstrated reduced heart rate, and blood pressure readings.

Lundeberg T (1984). Long-term results of vibratory stimulation as a pain relieving measure for chronic pain. *Pain* **20:13–23**

Method: 267 patients with chronic neurogenic or musculoskeletal pain were given vibratory stimulation for their pain. The patients were observed for 18 months or until they terminated the treatment.

Results: About half of the successfully relieved patients (59% of the total number of patients) reported more than 50% pain relief, as scored on a visual analog and an adjective scale. Seventy-two percent of these patients reported increased social activity and greater than 50% reported reduced intake of analgesic drugs after 12 months of home treatment.

Lundeberg T, Abrahamsson P, Bondesson L, et al (1987). Effect of vibratory stimulation on experimental and clinical pain. *Scandinavian Journal of Rehabilitation Medicine* **20:149–159**

Method: The effect of vibratory stimulation on experimental pain of the skin overlying the right and left extensor carpi radialis longus muscle induced by electrical stimulation was studied in 16 healthy subjects and in 18 patients suffering from chronic epicondyalgia of the right elbow.

Results: In the healthy subjects there were no side differences whereas in the patients, the skin pain threshold over the painful right muscle was lower than that of the left unaffected side under resting conditions. After vibratory stimulation, the skin pain threshold increased bilaterally by 1.1–1.6 times the pre-stimulation threshold in the healthy subjects and by 1.2–2.3 times this threshold in the patients. In eight of the healthy subjects there was an increase in peripheral blood flow during stimulation and in eight there was a small decrease. In 13 patients the change in pain threshold was seen in phase with the local increase and decrease in peripheral blood flow. In all individuals, the pain thresholds were regained within 45 minutes of cessation of stimulation. This was in contrast to the general subjective pain in the patients; 12 patients reported that the relief of pain lasted for a period of 1–7 hours.

Lundeberg T, Abrahamsson P, Haker E (1987). Vibratory stimulation compared to placebo in alleviation of pain. *Scandinavian Journal of Rehabilitation Medicine* **19:153–158**

Method: The placebo effect of vibratory stimulation was studied in 72 patients with chronic pain syndromes in a double-blind crossover trial using a vibrator and a 'placebo unit'.
Results: Pain alleviation was reported by 48% of the patients during vibratory stimulation compared with 34% for placebo treatment.

Mobily PR, Herr KA, Nicholson AC (1994). Validation of cutaneous stimulation for pain management. *International Journal of Nursing Studies* **31:533–544**

Method: The purpose of this study was to identify and validate pain management interventions including heat and cold application, massage and transcutaneous electrical nerve stimulation (TENS). A two-round Delphi survey was completed by nurses selected for their expertise in pain management.
Results: Data analyses revealed that consistently high scores were obtained by the raters for each intervention and activity.

Nixon M, Teschendorff J, Finney J, et al (1997). Expanding the nursing repertoire: the effect of massage on post-operative pain. *Australian Journal of Advanced Nursing* **14:21–26**

Method: A treatment group of 19 patients and a control group of 20 patients were compared on the impact of massage therapy on patients' perceptions of post-operative pain.
Results: Controlling for age, the results indicated that massage produced a significant reduction in patients' perceptions of pain over a 24-hour period.

Piotrowski MM, Paterson C, Mitchinson A, et al (2003). Massage as adjuvant therapy in the management of acute postoperative pain: a preliminary study in men. *Journal of the American College of Surgeons* **197:1037–1046**

Method: Opioid analgesia alone may not fully relieve all aspects of acute postoperative pain. Complementary medicine techniques used as adjuvant therapies have the potential to improve pain management and palliate post-operative distress.

Study design: This prospective randomized clinical trial compared pain relief after major operations in 202 patients who received one of three nursing interventions: massage, focused attention, or routine care. Interventions were performed twice daily starting 24 hours after the operation through post-operative day 7. Perceived pain was measured each morning.

Results: The rate of decline in the unpleasantness of postoperative pain was accelerated by massage ($p = 0.05$). Massage also accelerated the rate of decline in the intensity of postoperative pain but this effect was not statistically significant. Use of opioid analgesics was not altered significantly by the interventions.

Conclusions: Massage may be a useful adjuvant therapy for the management of acute postoperative pain. Its greatest effect appears to be on the affective component (i.e. unpleasantness) of the pain.

van den Dolder PA, Roberts DL (2003). A trial into the effectiveness of soft tissue massage in the treatment of shoulder pain. *The Australian Journal of Physiotherapy* **49:183–188**

Method: The purpose of this single blinded randomized controlled trial was to investigate the effects of soft tissue massage on range of motion, reported pain and reported function in patients with shoulder pain. Twenty-nine patients referred to physiotherapy for shoulder pain were randomly assigned to a treatment group that received six treatments of soft tissue massage around the shoulder (n = 15) or to a control group that received no treatment while on the waiting list for two weeks (n = 14). Measurements were taken both before and after the experimental period by a blinded assessor. Active range of motion was measured for flexion, abduction and hand-behind-back movements. Pain was assessed with the Short Form McGill Pain Questionnaire (SFMPQ) and functional ability was assessed with the Patient Specific Functional Disability Measure (PSFDM).

Results: The treatment group showed significant improvements in range of motion compared with the control group for abduction (mean 42.2°, 95% CI 24.1–60.4°), flexion (mean 22.6°, 95% CI 12.4–32.8°) and hand-behind-back (mean 11.0 cm improvement, 95% CI 6.3–15.6 cm). Massage reduced pain as reported on the descriptive section of the SFMPQ by a mean of 4.9 points (95% CI 2.5–7.2 points) and on the visual analog scale by an average of 26.5 mm (95% CI 5.3–47.6 mm), and it improved reported function on the PSFDM by a mean of 8.6 points (95% CI 4.9–12.3 points). We conclude that soft tissue massage around the shoulder is effective in improving range of motion, pain and function in patients with shoulder pain. The mechanisms behind these effects remain unclear.

Walach H, Guthlin C, Konig M (2003). Efficacy of massage therapy in chronic pain: a pragmatic randomized trial. *Journal of Alternative & Complementary Medicine* **9:837–846**

Method: Although classic massage is used widely in Germany and elsewhere for treating chronic pain conditions, there are no randomized controlled trials (RCT).

Design: Pragmatic RCT of classic massage compared to standard medical care (SMC) in chronic pain conditions of back, neck, shoulders, head and limbs.

Outcome measure: Pain rating (nine-point Likert-scale; predefined main outcome criterion) at pretreatment, post-treatment, and 3-month follow-up, as well as pain adjective list, depression, anxiety, mood, and body concept.

Results: Because of political and organizational problems, only 29 patients were randomized, 19 to receive massage, 10 to SMC. Pain improved significantly in both groups, but only in the massage group was it still significantly improved at follow-up. Depression and anxiety were improved significantly by both treatments, yet only in the massage group were maintained at follow-up. Despite its limitation resulting from problems with numbers and randomization this study shows that massage can be at least as effective as SMC in chronic pain syndromes. Relative changes are equal, but tend to last longer and to generalize more into psychologic domains. Because this is a pilot study, the results need replication, but our experiences might be useful for other researchers.

Wang HL, Keck JF (2004). Foot and hand massage as an intervention for postoperative pain. *Pain Management Nursing* **5:59–65**

Method: Physiological responses to pain create harmful effects that prolong the body's recovery after surgery. Patients routinely report mild-to-moderate pain even though pain medications have been administered. Complementary strategies based on sound research findings are needed to supplement post-operative pain relief using pharmacologic management. Foot and hand massage has the potential to assist in pain relief. Massaging the feet and hands stimulates the mechanoreceptors that activate the 'nonpainful' nerve fibers, preventing pain transmission from reaching consciousness. The purpose of this pretest–post-test design study was to investigate whether a 20-minute foot and hand massage (5 minutes to each extremity), which was provided 1–4 hours after a dose of pain medication, would reduce pain perception and sympathetic responses among postoperative patients. A convenience sample of 18 patients rated pain intensity and pain distress using a 0–10 numeric rating scale.

Results: Participants reported decreases in pain intensity from 4.65 to 2.35 ($t = 8.154$, $p < 0.001$) and in pain distress from 4.00 to 1.88 ($t = 5.683$, $p < 0.001$). Statistically significant decreases in sympathetic responses to pain (i.e. heart rate and respiratory rate) were observed although blood pressure remained unchanged. The changes in heart rate and respiratory rate were not clinically significant. The patients experienced moderate pain after they received pain medications. This pain was reduced by the intervention, thus supporting the effectiveness of massage in postoperative pain management. Foot and hand massage appears to be an effective, inexpensive, low-risk, flexible, and easily applied strategy for postoperative pain management.

PARKINSON'S DISEASE

Hernandez-Reif M, Field T, Largie S, et al (2002). Parkinson's disease symptoms are reduced by massage therapy and progressive muscle exercises. *Journal of Bodywork and Movement Therapies* 6:177–182

Method: Sixteen adults diagnosed with idiopathic Parkinson's disease (mean age = 58), received 30-minute massage therapy or progressive muscle relaxation sessions twice a week for five weeks (10 sessions total).

Results: Physicians rated massage therapy participants as improved in daily living activities by the end of the study. Participants also rated themselves as improved in daily functioning including having more effective and less disturbed sleep.

PERINEAL MASSAGE

Davidson K, Jacoby S, Brown MS (2000). Prenatal perineal massage: preventing lacerations during delivery. *Journal of Obstetric, Gynecologic, & Neonatal Nursing* 29:474–479

Method: This study investigated the associations between perineal lacerations and 13 variables associated with the incidence of perineal lacerations. 368 women were assessed.

Results: When parity was controlled, the only factors independently associated with the seriousness of lacerations were parity and prenatal perineal massage. Thus, this study supports the teaching of perineal massage.

Labrecque M, Marcoux S, Pinault JJ, et al (1994). Prevention of perineal trauma by perineal massage during pregnancy: a pilot study. *Birth* 21:20–25

Method: Although the performance of perineal massage by a woman or her partner during the last weeks of pregnancy may help to prevent perineal trauma at delivery, the technique has never been evaluated rigorously. This study examined the feasibility of a randomized, controlled trial, and more specifically assessed the participation rate, the acceptability of the intervention, and whether or not an attending physician could remain blind to the participants' groups. Thus, this pilot study was a single-blinded, randomized, controlled trial. Nulliparous women, 32–34 weeks pregnant, were recruited. Women assigned to the intervention group practiced daily 10-minute perineal massage and completed a diary, and those in the control group had standard care. Among the 174 women who delivered during the study period, 68% were approached by a midwife and 26% were randomized. 91% of the 22 women in the massage group returned their perineal massage diaries.

Research: Based on the postpartum questionnaire, 20 women practiced the technique at least four times a week for 3 weeks or longer. No woman in the control group practiced massage. The attending physician was aware of the woman's group in only 7% of cases. Based on the results of this pilot study, a randomized, controlled trial to evaluate the efficacy of perineal massage in preventing perineal trauma at birth appears feasible.

Labrecque M, Eason E, Marcoux S (2001). Women's views on the practice of prenatal perineal massage. *British Journal of Obstetrics & Gynaecology* **108:499–504**

Method: 763 women received perineal massage during pregnancy. Based on a factor analysis, 17 of the questions were classified into four categories: acceptability of perineal massage (eight items); preparation for birth (four items); relationship with the partner (two items); and effect of massage on delivery (three items). The last two questions asked whether women would perform the massage in their next pregnancy and whether they would recommend perineal massage to another pregnant woman.

Results: Pain and technical problems reported during the first week or two of massage tended to disappear after a few weeks. Women's assessment of the effect of massage on preparation for birth and on delivery was positive. Women's views about the effect on their relationship with their partner were either positive or negative and were proportional to the partner's participation with the massage. Most women said they would massage again if they were to have another pregnancy and would recommend it to another pregnant woman.

PHYSICAL ACTIVITY

Aly H, Moustafa MF, Hassanein SM, et al (2004). Physical activity combined with massage improves bone mineralization in the premature infants: a randomized trial. *Journal of Perinatology* **24:305–309**

Method: Osteopenia of prematurity is a known source for morbidity in preterm infants. Premature infants have shown favorable outcomes in response to massage and physical activity. Whether such intervention can stimulate bone formation or decrease bone resorption is yet to be determined.

Objective: To test the hypothesis that massage combined with physical activity can stimulate bone formation and ameliorate bone resorption in premature infants. A prospective double-blinded randomized trial was conducted at the Neonatal Intensive Care Unit of Ain Shams University in Cairo, Egypt. Thirty preterm infants (28–35 weeks' gestation) were randomly assigned to either control group (Group I, n = 15) or intervention group (Group II, n = 15). Infants in the intervention group received a daily protocol of combined massage and physical activity. Serum type I collagen C-terminal propeptide

(PICP) and urinary pyridinoline crosslinks of collagen (Pyd) were used as indices for bone formation and resorption, respectively. PICP and Pyd were measured at enrollment and at discharge for all subjects. T-test, ANOVA and linear regression analysis were used for statistical analyses.

Results: There was no difference between groups I and II in gestational age (32.1 +/−1.8 vs 31.5 +/−1.4 weeks) or birth weight (1.429 +/−0.148 vs 1.467 +/−0.132 g). In the control group, serum PICP decreased over time from 82.3+/−8.5 to 68.78 +/−14.6 ($p < 0.01$), while urinary Pyd increased from 447.7 +/−282.8 to 744.9 +/−373.6 ($p < 0.01$) indicating decreased bone formation and increased bone resorption, respectively. In the intervention group, serum PICP increased over time from 62.5 +/−13.8 to 73.84 +/−12.9 ($p < 0.01$). Urinary Pyd also increased over time from 445.7 +/−266.5 to 716.8 +/−301.8 ($p < 0.01$). In a linear regression model including gestational age and intervention, serum PICP increased significantly in the intervention group (regression coefficient 18.8 +/−4.6, $p = 0.0001$) while urinary Pyd did not differ between groups (regression coefficient = 5.6 +/−114.3, $p = 0.961$). A combined massage and physical activity protocol improved bone formation (PICP) but did not affect bone resorption (Pyd). Pyd increased over time in both groups, possibly due to continuous bone resorption and Ca mobilization.

PHYSIOLOGY

Delaney JP, Leong KS, Watkins A, et al (2002). The short-term effects of myofascial trigger point massage therapy on cardiac autonomic tone in healthy subjects. *Journal of Advanced Nursing* 37:364–371

Method: To investigate the effects of myofascial trigger-point massage therapy to the head, neck and shoulder areas on cardiac autonomic tone.

Background: No studies have reported on the effect of back massage on autonomic tone as measured by heart rate variability. This is especially relevant to the nursing profession, as massage is increasingly available as a therapy complementary to conventional nursing practice. An experimental study in which subjects were initially placed in age- and sex-matched groups and then randomized to treatment or control by alternate allocation. The study involved 30 healthy subjects (16 female and 14 male, aged 32.47 +/− 1.55 years, mean +/− standard error). A 5-minute cardiac interbeat interval recording, systolic and diastolic blood pressure and subjective self-evaluations of muscle tension and emotional state were taken before and after intervention. Autonomic function was measured using time and frequency domain analysis of heart rate variability.

Results: Following myofascial trigger-point massage therapy there was a significant decrease in heart rate ($p < 0.01$), systolic blood pressure ($p = 0.02$) and diastolic blood pressure ($p < 0.01$). Analysis of heart rate variability revealed a significant increase in parasympathetic activity ($p < 0.01$) following myofascial trigger-point massage therapy. Additionally both muscle tension and emotional state, showed significant improvement ($p < 0.01$).

Conclusions: In normal healthy subjects myofascial trigger-point massage therapy to the head, neck and shoulder areas is effective in increasing cardiac parasympathetic activity and improving measures of relaxation.

Diego MA, Field T, Sanders C, et al (2004). Massage therapy of moderate and light pressure and vibrator effects on EEG and heart rate. *International Journal of Neuroscience* **114:31–44**

Method: Three types of commonly used massage therapy techniques were assessed in a sample of 36 healthy adults, randomly assigned to: (1) moderate massage, (2) light massage, or (3) vibratory stimulation group (n = 12 per group). Changes in anxiety and stress were assessed, and EEG and EKG were recorded.

Results: Anxiety scores decreased for all groups, but the moderate pressure massage group reported the greatest decrease in stress. The moderate massage group also experienced a decrease in heart rate and EEG changes including an increase in delta and a decrease in alpha and beta activity, suggesting a relaxation response. Finally, this group showed increased positive affect, as indicated by a shift toward left frontal EEG activation. The light massage group showed increased arousal, as indicated by decreased delta and increased beta activity and increased heart rate. The vibratory stimulation group also showed increased arousal, as indicated by increased heart rate and increased theta, alpha, and beta activity.

POSTBURN

Field T, Peck M, Hernandez-Reif, M, et al (2000). Postburn itching, pain, and psychological symptoms are reduced with massage therapy. *Journal of Burn Care & Rehabilitation* **21:189–193**

Method: Twenty patients with burn injuries were randomly assigned to a massage therapy or a standard treatment control group during the remodeling phase of wound healing. The massage therapy group received a 30-minute massage with cocoa butter to a closed, moderate-sized scar tissue area twice a week for 5 weeks.

Results: The massage therapy group reported reduced itching, pain, and anxiety and improved mood immediately after the first and last therapy sessions, and their ratings on these measures improved from the first day to the last day of the study.

POST-TRAUMATIC STRESS DISORDER

Field T, Seligman S, Scafidi F, et al (1996). Alleviating posttraumatic stress in children following Hurricane Andrew. *Journal of Applied Developmental Psychology* **17:37–50**

Method: Massage therapy was evaluated for the reduction of anxiety and depression in children as measured by behavioral observations, their drawings, and their cortisol levels. Sixty 1st–5th graders who showed classroom behavior problems following Hurricane Andrew were randomly assigned to a massage therapy or a video attention control group.

Results: Scores on the Post-traumatic Stress Disorder Index suggest that the subjects were experiencing severe post-traumatic stress. Subjects who received massage reported being happier and less anxious and had lower salivary cortisol levels after the therapy than the video subjects. The massage group showed more sustained changes as manifested by lower scores on anxiety and depression scales and on self-drawings. The massage therapy subjects were also observed to be more relaxed.

PREGNANCY

Field T, Hernandez-Reif M, Hart S, et al (1999). Pregnant women benefit from massage therapy. *Journal of Psychosomatic Obstetrics & Gynecology* **20:31–38**

Method: Twenty-six pregnant women were assigned to a massage therapy or a relaxation therapy group for 5 weeks. The therapies consisted of 20-minute sessions twice a week.

Results: Both groups reported feeling less anxious after the first session and less leg pain after the first and last sessions. Only the massage therapy group, however, reported reduced anxiety, improved mood, better sleep and less back pain by the last day of the study. In addition, urinary stress hormone levels (norepinephrine) decreased for the massage therapy group, and the women had fewer complications during labor, and their infants had fewer postnatal complications (e.g. less prematurity).

Norheim AJ, Pederson EJ, Fonnebo V, et al (2001). Acupressure treatment of morning sickness in pregnancy. A randomized, double-blind, placebo-controlled study. *Scandinavian Journal of Primary Health Care* **19:43–47**

Method: To find out whether acupressure wristband can alleviate nausea and vomiting in early pregnancy.

Design: Double-blind, placebo-controlled study.

Subjects: 97 women with mean gestational length completed 8–12 weeks.

Main outcome measures: Symptoms were recorded according to intensity, duration and nature of complaints.

Results: 71% of women in the intervention group reported both less intensive morning sickness and reduced duration of symptoms. The same tendency was seen in the placebo group, with 59% reporting less intensity and 63% shorter duration of symptoms. However, a significance level of 5% was reached only in the case of duration of symptoms, which was reduced by 2.74 hours in the intervention group compared to 0.85 hours in the placebo group ($p = 0.018$).

Conclusions: Acupressure wristband might be an alternative therapy for morning sickness in early pregnancy, especially before pharmaceutical treatment is considered.

Werntoft E, Dykes AK (2001). Effect of acupressure on nausea and vomiting during pregnancy. A randomized, placebo-controlled, pilot study. *Journal of Reproductive Medicine* **46:835–839**

Method: To compare the antiemetic effect of acupressure at the Neiguan point (P6) in a group of healthy women with normal pregnancy and nausea and vomiting during pregnancy (NVP) with a similar group receiving acupressure at a placebo point and another, similar group not receiving any treatment.
Study design: A randomized, placebo-controlled, pilot study involving 60 women.
Results: It is possible to reduce NVP significantly with acupressure at P6 as compared to acupressure at a placebo point or no treatment at all in healthy women with normal pregnancies. Relief from nausea appeared 1 day after starting treatment in both the P6 and placebo groups but lasted for only 6 days in the placebo group. The P6 group, however, experienced significantly less nausea after 14 days as compared to the other two groups.
Conclusion: This study involved 60 healthy women with normal pregnancy and suffering from NVP. According to the results, in healthy women with normal pregnancy it is possible to reduce NVP significantly at P6 as compared to acupressure at a placebo point and to no treatment.

PREMENSTRUAL SYNDROME

Hernandez-Reif M, Martinez A, Field T, et al (2000). Premenstrual syndrome symptoms are relieved by massage therapy. *Journal of Psychosomatic Obstetrics & Gynecology* **21:9–15**

Method: Twenty-four women with premenstrual syndrome were randomly assigned to a massage therapy or a relaxation therapy group.
Results: The massage group showed decreases in anxiety, depressed mood and pain immediately after the massage sessions. In addition, by the last day of the study the massage therapy group reported a reduction in menstrual distress symptoms including pain and water retention. These data suggest that massage therapy is effective for treating premenstrual syndrome.

PRESCHOOL MASSAGE

Field T, Kilmer T, Hernandez-Reif M, et al (1996). Preschool children's sleep and wake behavior: effects of massage therapy. *Early Child Development and Care* **120:39–44**

Method: Preschool children received 20-minute massages twice a week for 5 weeks.
Results: The massaged children as compared to children in the wait-list control group had better behavior ratings on state, vocalization, activity and cooperation after the massage sessions on the first and last days of the study. Their behavior was also rated more optimally by their teachers by the end of the study. Also, at the end of the 5-week period parents of the massaged

children rated their children as having less touch aversion and being more extroverted. Finally, the massaged children had a shorter latency to naptime sleep by the end of the study.

Hart S, Field T, Hernandez-Reif M, et al (1998). Preschoolers' cognitive performance improves following massage. *Early Child Development and Care* **143:59–64**

Method: Examined the effects of massage therapy on the cognitive performance of preschool students. 20 preschool students (aged 3.3–5.5 years) were rated by their teacher on a temperament checklist. Additionally, subjects completed the Block Design, Animal Pegs, and Mazes subtests of the Wechsler Preschool and Primary Scale of Intelligence (WPPSI) prior to and following some subjects receiving a 15-minute massage.

Results: Subjects' scores on the Block Design test of abstract reasoning improved following massage. In contrast, scores of control subjects did not improve. On the Animal Pegs matching task, subjects maintained the levels of accuracy they had shown on the pretest, while control subjects became less accurate. Massage was particularly beneficial to subjects rated as high-strung and anxious. Compared with subjects rated by their teachers as calm and easygoing, anxious subjects showed greater improvements on the Block Design and maintained greater accuracy on Animal Pegs subtests.

PRETERM INFANTS

Dieter JNI (1999). The effects of tactile/kinesthetic stimulation on the physiology and behavior of preterm infants. *Dissertation Abstracts International: Section B–The Sciences and Engineering* **60:23–35**

Method: This study examined the effects of 10 days of preterm infant tactile/kinesthetic stimulation (T/K: massage and limb flexion–extension) on state and motor behavior, heart and respiration rate, cardiac vagal tone (CVT), weight gain, and neurobehavioral adaptation. Medically stable 'grower nursery' infants were randomly assigned to the T/K (n = 15) and control (n = 15) groups.

Results: During T/K, infants showed higher heart rates and CVT, increased yawning, crying, vocalizations, active sleep, multiple limb and gross body movements than observed during baseline. These effects did not diminish over the 10 days. No difference was found in heart and respiration rates when T/K was compared to physical exams/diaper changes. T/K infants exhibited higher heart rates than control infants prior to and during physical exams/diaper changes. T/K infants demonstrated greater weight gain than control infants during the first week. Curve estimate analyses revealed a linear relationship between the amount of time an infant spent in the quiet alert state during T/K and subsequent weight gain. A quadratic relationship was found between CVT during T/K and total week 1 weight gain. No group differences were observed in formula and kilocalorie intake. T/K infants exhibited a greater volumetric output and number of bowel movements than control infants. T/K infants were more alert during bottle-feeding than control infants. The duration of bottle feeds was longer for T/K infants than for control infants.

Dieter JNI, Field T, Hernandez-Reif M, et al (2003). Stable preterm infants gain more weight and sleep less after five days of massage therapy. *Journal of Pediatric Psychology* **28:403–411**

Method: To determine whether a shorter course of massage therapy leads to greater weight gain in grower nursery preterm infants, massage therapy (body stroking and passive limb movement for three 15-minute periods per day for 5 days) was provided for 14 preterm neonates (mean gestational age, 30.2 weeks; mean birthweight, 1215 g) and their weight gain, formula intake, kilocalories, and stooling, were compared with a group of 14 control infants (mean gestational age, 31.3 weeks; mean birthweight, 1392 g).
Results: Massaged infants gained 47% more weight per day than control infants, (Massage mean = 37.1 g; Control mean = 25.2 g). No significant group differences were found in formula and kilocalorie intake, stooling, or number of family visits during participation.

Ferber SG, Kuint J, Weller A, et al (2002). Massage therapy by mothers and trained professionals enhances weight gain in preterm infants. *Early Human Development* **37:37–45**

Method: This study replicated the results of increased weight gain in the course of 'massage therapy' in preterm infants, and utilized a new, cost-effective application of this method by comparing maternal to nonmaternal administration of the therapy. The study comprised 57 healthy, preterm infants assigned to three groups: two treatment groups—one in which the mothers performed the massage, and the other in which a professional female unrelated to the infant administered the treatment. Both these groups were compared to a control group.
Results: Over the 10-day study period, the two treatment groups gained significantly more weight compared to the control group (291.3 and 311.3 vs 225.5 g, respectively). Calorie intake/kg did not differ between groups.

Field T (2001). Massage therapy facilitates weight gain in preterm infants. *Current Directions in Psychological Science* **10:51–54**

Review: Studies from several labs have documented a 31–47% greater weight gain in preterm newborns receiving massage therapy (three 15-minute sessions for 5–10 days) compared with standard medical treatment. Although the underlying mechanism for this relationship between massage therapy and weight gain has not yet been established, possibilities that have been explored in studies with both humans and rats include (a) increased protein synthesis, (b) increased vagal activity that releases food-absorption hormones like insulin and enhances gastric motility and (c) decreased cortisol levels leading to increased oxytocin. In addition, functional magnetic resonance imaging studies are being conducted to assess the effects of touch therapy on brain development. Further behavioral, physiological, and genetic research is needed to understand these effects of massage therapy on growth and development.

Field T, Schanberg SM (1990). Massage alters growth and catecholamine production in preterm newborns. In: Gunzenhauser N, Brazelton TB, Field T (eds) Johnson & Johnson. Advances in touch. *Skillman, NJ,* **pp 85–97**

Method: Forty medically stable preterm nenonates received tactile/kinesthetic stimulation for three 15-minute periods during 3 consecutive hours every day for 10 days.

Results: Despite similar formula and caloric intake, the treatment infants averaged a 21% greater daily weight gain than the control infants over the treatment. In addition, the treatment group showed superior performance on the NBAS on the habituation cluster following the treatment period, and less time in active sleep and less facial grimacing, mouthing/yawning, and clenched fists.

Field T, Schanberg S, Scafidi F, et al (1986). Tactile/kinesthetic stimulation effects on preterm neonates. *Pediatrics* **77:654–658**

Method: Tactile/kinesthetic stimulation was given to 20 preterm neonates (mean gestational age, 31 weeks; mean birth weight, 1280 g; mean time in neonatal intensive care unit, 20 days) during transitional ('grower') nursery care, and their growth, sleep–wake behavior, and Brazelton scale performance was compared with a group of 20 control neonates. The tactile/kinesthetic stimulation consisted of body stroking and passive movements of the limbs for three, 15-minute periods per day for 10 days.

Results: The stimulated neonates averaged a 47% greater weight gain per day (mean 25 g vs 17 g), were more active and alert during sleep/wake behavior observations, and showed more mature habituation, orientation, motor, and range of state behavior on the Brazelton scale than control infants. Finally, their hospital stay was 6 days shorter, yielding a cost saving of approximately $3000 per infant. These data suggest that tactile/kinesthetic stimulation may be a cost-effective way of facilitating growth and behavioral organization even in very small preterm neonates.

Jones E, Dimmock PW, Spencer SA (2001). A randomised controlled trial to compare methods of milk expression after preterm delivery. *Archives of Disease in Childhood Fetal & Neonatal Edition* **85:F91–95**

Method: The objective of this study was to compare sequential and simultaneous breast pumping on volume of milk expressed and its fat content. Thirty-six women were analyzed; 19 women used simultaneous pumping and 17 used sequential pumping. Women were randomly allocated to use either simultaneous (both breasts simultaneously) or sequential (one breast then the other) milk expression. Stratification was used to ensure that the groups were balanced for parity and gestation. A crossover design was used for massage, with patients acting as their own controls. Women were randomly allocated to receive either massage or non-massage first.

Results: Milk yield per expression was: sequential pumping with no massage, 51.32 g (95% confidence interval (CI) 56.57–46.07); sequential pumping with massage, 78.71 g (95% CI 85.19–72.24); simultaneous pumping with no massage, 87.69 g (95% CI 96.80–78.57); simultaneous pumping with massage, 125.08 g (95% CI 140.43–109.74). The fat concentration in the milk was not affected by the increase in volume achieved by the interventions.

Kuhn C, Schanberg S, Field T, et al (1991). Tactile kinesthetic stimulation effects on sympathetic and adrenocortical function in preterm infants. *Journal of Pediatrics* **119:434–440**

Method: The purpose of this study was to investigate the neuroendocrine response in preterm infants to a pattern of tactile-kinesthetic stimulation that facilitates their growth and development. Preterm infants (mean gestational age 30 weeks, mean birth weight 1176 g) received normal nursery care or tactile-kinesthetic stimulation for three 15-minute periods at the start of three consecutive hours each day for 10 days. On day 1 and day 10 of the study, a 24-hour urine sample was collected for norepinephrine, epinephrine, dopamine, cortisol, and creatinine assay and a blood sample was taken by heel stick for cortisol and growth hormone assay.

Results: Urine norepinephrine and epinephrine values increased significantly only in the stimulated babies. Urine dopamine and cortisol values increased in both groups, and serum growth hormone decreased in both groups. Individual differences in urine norepinephrine, epinephrine, dopamine, and cortisol values were highly stable across the 10 days despite a 10-fold range of values among the infants. The results of this study suggest that tactile-kinesthetic stimulation of preterm infants has a fairly specific effect on maturation and/or activity of the sympathetic nervous system. In addition, this study has defined catecholamine and cortisol secretion across gestational age in normal preterm infants. Finally, these data suggest that highly stable individual levels of catecholamine and cortisol secretion are established by birth in humans.

Mathai S, Fernandez A, Mondkar J, et al (2002). Effects of tactile-kinesthetic stimulation in preterms: a controlled trial. *Indian Pediatrics* **38:1091–1098**

Method: The objective of this study was to determine the effects of tactile-kinesthetic stimulation on preterms on physiologic parameters, physical growth and behavioral development. Forty-eight well preterms with birth weights between 1000 and 2000 g were randomly assigned to treatment and control groups. Treatment babies received tactile-kinesthetic stimulation in the form of a structured baby massage from day 3 to term-corrected age. They were observed for changes in vital parameters (heart rate, respiration, temperature and oxygen saturation) during the first few days of stimulation in hospital. Thereafter, massage was continued at home. Changes in weight, length and head circumference and neuro-behavior (Brazelton Neuro-Behavioral Assessment Scale) were assessed in both groups before, during and after the study period.

Results: An increase in heart rate (within physiologic range) was seen in the treatment group during stimulation. This group also showed a weight gain of 4.24 g/day more than controls. On the Brazelton Scale the massaged group showed improved scores on the 'orientation', 'range of state', 'regulation of state' and 'autonomic stability' clusters at follow-up.

Morrow CJ, Field T, Scafidi FA, et al (1991). Differential effects of massage and heelstick procedures on transcutaneous oxygen tension in preterm neonates. *Infant Behavior and Development* **14:397–414**

Method: This study investigated the effects of heelsticks and tactile-kinesthetic massage on transcutaneous oxygen tension ($TcPO_2$) in 47 stabilized preterm neonates (average gestational age 30 weeks).

Results: During the heelstick procedure, $TcPO_2$ significantly declined an average of 14 mmHg. When compared with the tactile-kinesthetic massage, $TcPO_2$ levels during the heelstick were significantly lower than during the stimulation. Mean $TcPO_2$ levels remained clinically safe during the four massage sessions. The $TcPO_2$ levels during kinesthetic stimulation were somewhat more varied, and movement and pressurization of the $TcPO_2$ electrode were investigated as possible artifactual explanations for this phenomenon. Overall, findings indicate that social forms of touch such as tactile-kinesthetic massage do not appear to have a medically compromising effect on $TcPO_2$ in the preterm neonate. Findings are evaluated in relation to the 'minimal touch' policy.

Scafidi F, Field T, Schanberg S, et al (1986). Effects of tactile/kinesthetic stimulation on the clinical course and sleep/wake behavior of preterm neonates. *Infant Behavior and Development* **9:91–105**

Method: Forty preterm neonates treated in an intensive care nursery (mean gestational age = 31 weeks, mean birthweight = 1274 g) were randomly assigned to a treatment or control group. The treatment infants received tactile/kinesthetic stimulation (body massage and passive movements of the limbs) for three 15-minute periods during three consecutive hours for a 10-day period. At the end of the treatment period the behavioral states and activity level of the neonates were monitored during sleep/wake behavior observations. In addition, neonatal behaviors were assessed on the Brazelton scale.

Results: The treated infants averaged a 47% greater weight gain per day (25 vs 17 g), and spent more time awake and active during sleep/wake behavior observations. On the Brazelton scale the treated infants showed more mature orientation, motor, habituation, and range of state behaviors. Finally, the treated infants were discharged 6 days earlier, yielding hospital cost savings of $3000 per infant.

Scafidi FA, Field TM, Schanberg SM, et al (1990). Massage stimulates growth in preterm infants: a replication. *Infant Behavior and Development* **13:167–188**

Method: Forty preterm infants (mean gestational age = 30 weeks; mean birthweight = 1176 g; mean duration ICU care = 14 days) were assigned to treatment and control groups once they were considered medically stable. Assignments were based on a random stratification of gestational age, birthweight, intensive care duration, and study entrance weight. The treatment infants (n = 20) received tactile/kinesthetic stimulation for three 15-minute periods during 3 consecutive hours per day for a 10-day period. Sleep/wake behavior was monitored and Brazelton assessments were performed at the beginning and at the end of the treatment period.

Results: The treated infants averaged a 21% greater weight gain per day (34 vs 28 g) and were discharged 5 days earlier. No significant differences were demonstrated in sleep/wake states and activity level between the groups. The treated infants' performance was superior on the habituation cluster items of the Brazelton scale. Finally, the treatment infants were more active during the stimulation sessions than during the nonstimulation observation sessions (particularly during the tactile segments of the sessions).

Scafidi FA, Field T, Schanberg SM (1993). Factors that predict which preterm infants benefit most from massage therapy. *Journal of Developmental & Behavioral Pediatrics* **14:176–180**

Method: Ninety-three preterm infants (mean gestational age = 30 weeks; mean birthweight = 1204 g; mean ICU duration = 15 days) were randomly assigned to a massage therapy group or a control group once they were considered medically stable. The treatment group (n = 50) received three daily 15-minute massages for 10 days.

Results: The massage therapy infants gained more weight per day (32 vs 29 g) than the control infants. The treatment and control groups were divided into high and low weight gainers based on the average weight gain for the control group. 70% of the massage therapy infants were classified as high weight gainers whereas only 40% of the control infants were classified as high weight gainers. Discriminant function analyses determining the characteristics that distinguished the high from the low weight gainers suggested that the control infants who, before the study, consumed more calories and spent less time in intermediate care gained more weight. In contrast, for the massage therapy group, the pattern of greater caloric intake and more days in intermediate care before the study period along with more obstetric complications differentiated the high from the low weight gainers, suggesting that the infants who had experienced more complications before the study benefited more from the massage therapy. These variables accurately predicted 78% of the infants who benefited more from the massage therapy.

Wheeden A, Scafidi FA, Field T, et al (1993). Massage effects on cocaine-exposed preterm neonates. *Journal of Developmental & Behavioral Pediatrics* **14:318–322**

Method: Thirty preterm cocaine-exposed preterm neonates (mean gestational age 30 weeks, mean birth weight = 1212 g, mean intensive care unit duration = 18 days) were randomly assigned to a massage therapy or a control group as soon as they were considered medically stable. Group assignment was based on a random stratification of gestational age, birth weight, intensive care unit duration, and entry weight into the study. The treatment group (n = 15) received massages for three 15-minute periods over three consecutive hours for a 10-day period.

Results: Findings suggested that the massaged infants (1) averaged 28% greater weight gain per day (33 vs 26 g) although the groups did not differ in intake (calories or volume), (2) showed significantly fewer postnatal complications and stress behaviors than did control infants, and (3) demonstrated more mature motor behaviors on the Brazelton examination at the end of the 10-day study period.

Whipple J (2000). The effect of parent training in music and multimodal stimulation on parent–neonate interactions in the neonatal intensive care unit. *Journal of Music Therapy* **37:250–268**

Methods: This study examined the effects of parent training in music and multimodal stimulation on the quantity and quality of parent–neonate interactions and the weight gain and length of hospitalization of premature and low birthweight (LBW) infants in a Neonatal Intensive Care Unit (NICU). Twenty sets of parents and premature LBW infants participated in the study. Parents in the experimental group received approximately 1 hour of instruction in appropriate uses of music, multimodal stimulation including massage techniques, and signs of infant overstimulation and techniques for its avoidance. Parent–neonate interactions, specifically parent actions and responses and infant stress and non-stress behaviors, were observed for subjects in both groups

Results: Infant stress behaviors were significantly fewer and appropriateness of parent actions and responses were significantly greater for experimental infants and parents than for control subjects. Parents in the experimental group also reported spending significantly more time visiting in the NICU than did parents of control infants.

PULMONARY DISEASE

Wu HS, Wu SC, Lin JG, et al (2004). Effectiveness of acupressure in improving dyspnoea in chronic obstructive pulmonary disease. *Journal of Advanced Nursing* 45:252–259

Method: Patients with chronic obstructive pulmonary disease (COPD) suffer from dyspnoea in their daily life and this may be increased by anxiety. Acupressure may promote relaxation and relieve dyspnoea. Thus, it is appropriate to explore the effectiveness of acupressure on dyspnoea in patients with COPD.

Aims: To compare outcomes of acupressure using sham acupoints on different meridians and ganglionic sections with that using true acupoints, in patients with COPD who are living at home. Patients diagnosed with COPD were selected from a medical center and three regional hospitals in Taipei. A randomized block experimental design was used. Using age, sex, pulmonary function, smoking, and steroid use as matching factors, 44 patients were randomly assigned either to a true acupoint acupressure or a sham group. The true acupoint acupressure group received a program to decrease dyspnoea. Those in the sham group received acupressure using sham pressure points. Both acupressure programs consisted of five sessions per week lasting 16 minutes per session, extending over 4 weeks for a total of 20 sessions. Before acupressure was initiated and at the conclusion of the 20th session, the Pulmonary Functional Status and Dyspnoea Questionnaire-modified scale and the Spielberger State Anxiety scale were administered, and a 6-minute walking distance test was performed. Physiological indicators of oxygen saturation and respiratory rate were measured before and after every session.

Results: Pulmonary function and dyspnoea scores, 6-minute walking distance measurements, state anxiety scale scores, and physiological indicators of the true acupoint acupressure group improved significantly compared with those of the sham group. The findings suggest that acupressure can be used as a nursing intervention to improve dyspnoea in patients with COPD.

REFLEXOLOGY

Kesselring A (1994). Fussreflexzonenmassage. *Schweizerische Medizinische Wochenschrift - Supplementum* 62:88–93

Foot reflexology is defined as massage of zones on the feet which correspond to different parts of the body. A Medline search yielded no literature in the field of foot reflexology. Indications for and results of foot reflexology have been extrapolated from case-descriptions and two pilot studies with small samples. One study (Lafuente et al) found foot reflexology to be as helpful to patients with headaches as medication (flunarizine), yet foot reflexology was fraught with fewer side-effects than medication. In a second study (Eichelberger et al) foot reflexology was used postoperatively on gynecological patients. The intervention group showed a lesser need for medication to enhance bladder tonus than did the control group. The literature describes foot reflexology as enhancing urination, bowel movements, and relaxation.

RENAL DISEASE

Tsay SL, Rong JR, Lin PF (2003). Acupoints massage in improving the quality of sleep and quality of life in patients with end-stage renal disease. *Journal of Advanced Nursing* **42:134–142**

Method: Traditional Chinese acupressure is a noninvasive technique that employs pressure and massage to acupoints in order to stimulate the balance of life energy that promotes health and comfort. Sleep disturbance is common in patients with end-stage renal disease but no intervention studies have addressed this problem. The purpose of the present study was to test the effectiveness of acupoints massage for patients with end-stage renal disease and experiencing sleep disturbances and diminished quality of life. The study was a randomized control trial. A total of 98 end-stage renal disease patients with sleep disturbances were randomly assigned into an acupressure group, a sham acupressure group, and a control group. Acupressure and sham acupressure group patients received acupoints or no acupoints massage three times a week during hemodialysis treatment for a total of 4 weeks. The measures included the Pittsburgh Sleep Quality Index, Sleep Log, and the Medical Outcome Study - Short Form 36.
Results: Their were significant differences between the acupressure group and the control group in Pittsburgh Sleep Quality Index subscale scores of subjective sleep quality, sleep duration, habitual sleep efficiency, sleep sufficiency, and global Pittsburgh Sleep Quality Index scores. Sleep log data revealed that the acupressure group significantly decreased wake time and experienced an improved quality of sleep at night over the control group. Medical Outcome Study - Short Form 36 data also documented that acupressure group patients experienced significantly improved quality of life.
Conclusion: This study supports the effectiveness of acupoints massage in improving the quality of sleep and life quality of end-stage renal disease patients, and offers a noninvasive therapy for sleep-disturbed patients.

REVIEWS

Field T (1998). Massage therapy effects. *American Psychologist* **53:1270–1281**

Review: Massage therapy is older than recorded time, and rubbing was the primary form of medicine until the pharmaceutical revolution of the 1940s. Popularized again as part of the alternative medicine movement, massage therapy has recently received empirical support for facilitating growth, reducing pain, increasing alertness, diminishing depression, and enhancing immune function. In this article studies are reviewed that document these effects, and models are proposed for potential underlying mechanisms.

Goats GC (1994). Massage—the scientific basis of an ancient art: Part 2. Physiological and therapeutic effects. [Review]. *British Journal of Sports Medicine* **28:153–156**

The physiological and therapeutic effects of massage are frequently questioned. This article reviews previous research on the effects of massage on blood flow and composition, edema, connective tissue, muscle and the nervous system. Although further investigations are clearly required in certain areas, the discussion demonstrates that the use of massage in sports medicine can be justified according to orthodox scientific criteria.

SEXUAL ABUSE

Field T, Hernandez-Reif M, Hart S, et al (1997). Sexual abuse effects are lessened by massage therapy. *Journal of Bodywork and Movement Therapies* **1:65–69**

Method: Women (mean age = 35 years) who had experienced sexual abuse, were given a 30-minute massage twice a week for 1 month.
Result: Immediately after the massage the women reported being less depressed and less anxious and their salivary cortisol levels decreased following the session. Over the 1-month treatment period the massage therapy group experienced a decrease in depression and in life event stress. Although the relaxation therapy control group also reported a decrease in anxiety and depression, their stress hormones did not change, and they reported an increasingly negative attitude toward touch.

SLEEP

Field T, Kilmer T, Hernandez-Reif M, et al (2002). Preschool children's sleep and wake behavior: effects of massage therapy. *Early Child Development and Care* **120:39–44**

Method: Preschool children received 20-minute massages twice a week for 5 weeks.
Results: The massaged children as compared to the children in the wait-list control group had better behavior ratings on state, vocalization, activity and cooperation after the massage sessions on the first and last days of the study. Their behavior was also rated more optimally by their teachers by the end of the study. Also, at the end of the 5-week period parents of the massaged children rated their children as having less touch aversion and being more extroverted. Finally, the massaged children had a shorter latency to naptime sleep by the end of the study.

Richards KC (1998). Effect of a back massage and relaxation intervention on sleep in critically ill patients. *American Journal of Critical Care* **7:288–299**

Method: Critically ill patients are deprived of sleep and its potential healing qualities, although many receive medications to promote sleep. This study determined the effects of (1) a back massage and (2) combined muscle relaxation, mental imagery, and a music audiotape on the sleep of older men with a cardiovascular illness who were hospitalized in a critical care unit. Sixty-nine subjects were randomly assigned to a 6-minute back massage (n = 24); a teaching session on relaxation and a 7.5-minute audiotape at bedtime consisting of muscle relaxation, mental imagery, and relaxing background music (n = 28); or the usual nursing care (controls, n = 17). Polysomnography was used to measure one night of sleep for each patient and the sleep efficiency index was the primary variable of interest.

Results: The analyses showed improved quality of sleep in the back-massage group.

SMOKING

Hernandez-Reif M, Field T, Hart S (1999). Smoking cravings are reduced by self-massage. *Preventive Medicine* **28:28–32**

Method: Attempts at smoking cessation have been correlated with severe withdrawal symptoms, including intense cigarette cravings, anxiety, and depressed mood. Massage therapy has been shown to reduce anxiety and stress hormones and improve mood. Twenty smokers were randomly assigned to a self-massage treatment or a control group. The treatment group was taught to conduct a hand or ear self-massage during three cravings a day for 1 month.

Results: Self-reports revealed lower anxiety scores, improved mood, and fewer withdrawal symptoms. In addition, the self-massage group smoked fewer cigarettes per day by the last week of the study. These findings suggest that self-massage may be an effective treatment for attempting smoking cessation, to alleviate smoking-related anxiety, reduce cravings and withdrawal symptoms, improve mood, and reduce the number of cigarettes smoked.

SPINAL CORD INJURIES

Diego MA, Field T, Hernandez-Reif M, et al (2002). Spinal cord patients benefit from massage therapy. *International Journal of Neuroscience* **112:133–142**

Method: This study assessed the effects of massage therapy on depression, functionality and upper body muscle strength and range of motion in spinal cord injury patients. Twenty spinal cord injury individuals recruited from a medical school outpatient clinic were randomly assigned to a massage therapy or a control group. Patients in the massage therapy group received two-40-

minute massage therapy sessions per week for 5 weeks. Patients in the control group practiced a range of motion exercise routines targeting the arms, neck, shoulders and back two times per week for 5 weeks.

Results: Although both the massage and exercise group appeared to benefit from treatment, only the massage group showed lower anxiety and depression scores and significantly increased muscle strength and wrist range of motion.

SPORTS

Smith LL, Keating MN, Holbert D, et al (1994). The effects of athletic massage on delayed onset muscle soreness, creatine kinase, and neutrophil count: a preliminary report. *Journal of Orthopaedic & Sports Physical Therapy* **19:93–99**

Method: It was hypothesized that athletic massage administered 2 hours after eccentric exercise would disrupt an initial crucial event in acute inflammation, the accumulation of neutrophils. This would result in a diminished inflammatory response and a concomitant reduction in delayed onset muscle soreness (DOMS) and serum creatine kinase (CK). Untrained males were randomly assigned to a massage (n = 7) or control (n = 7) group. All performed five sets of isokinetic eccentric exercise of the elbow flexors and extensors. Two hours after exercise, massage subjects received a 30-minute athletic massage; control subjects rested. Delayed onset muscle soreness and CK were assessed before exercise and at 8, 24, 48, 72, 96, and 120 hours after exercise. Circulating neutrophils were assessed before and immediately after exercise, and at 30-minute intervals for 8 hours; cortisol was assessed before and immediately after exercise, and at 30-minute intervals for 8 hours.

Results: Data analysis revealed a treatment effect for (1) DOMS, with the massage group reporting reduced levels; (2) CK, with the massage group displaying reduced levels; (3) neutrophils, with the massage group displaying a prolonged elevation; and (4) cortisol, with the massage group showing a diminished diurnal reduction.

Tiidus PM, Shoemaker JK (1995). Effleurage massage, muscle blood flow and long-term post-exercise strength recovery. *International Journal of Sports Medicine* **16:478–483**

Method: Manual massage is commonly assumed to enhance long-term muscle recovery from intense exercise, partly due to its ability to speed healing via enhanced muscle blood flow. We tested these assumptions by daily (for 4 days) massaging the quadriceps muscles of one leg on subjects who had previously completed an intense bout of eccentric quadriceps work with both legs.

Results: Immediate post-exercise isometric and dynamic quadriceps peak torque measures had declined to approximately 60–70% of pre-exercise values in both legs. Peak torques for both the massage and control leg tended to slowly return toward pre-exercise values through the subsequent 4 days (96 hours). There was no significant difference between the isometric and dynamic peak torques between massage and control legs up to 96 hours post-exercise. Leg blood flow was estimated by determining femoral artery and vein mean blood velocities via pulsed Doppler ultrasound velocimetry. Massage of the quadriceps muscles did not significantly elevate arterial or venous mean blood velocity above resting levels, while light quadriceps muscle contractions did. The perceived level of delayed onset muscle soreness tended to be reduced in the massaged leg 48–96 hours post-exercise. It was concluded that massage was not an effective treatment modality for enhancing long-term restoration of post-exercise muscle strength and its use for this purpose in athletic settings should be questioned

Viitasalo JT, Niemela K, Kaappola R, et al (1995). Warm underwater water-jet massage improves recovery from intense physical exercise. European *Journal of Applied Physiology & Occupational Physiology* **71:431–438**

Method: The effects of warm underwater water-jet massage on neuromuscular functioning, selected biochemical parameters (serum creatine kinase, lactic dehydrogenase, serum carbonic anhydrase, myoglobin, urine urea and creatinine) and muscle soreness were studied among 14 junior track and field athletes. Each subject spent, in a randomized order, two identical training weeks engaged in five strength/power training sessions lasting 3 days.
Results: The training weeks differed from each other only in respect of underwater water-jet massage treatments. These were used three times (20 minutes each) during the treatment week and not used during the control week. During the treatment week continuous jumping power decreased and ground contact time increased significantly less and serum myoglobin increased more than during the control week. It is suggested that underwater water-jet massage in connection with intense strength/power training increases the release of proteins from muscle tissue into the blood and enhances the maintenance of neuromuscular performance capacity.

STRESS

Meaney MJ, Aitken DH, Bhatnagar S, et al (1990). Neonatal handling and the development of the adrenocorticol response to stress. In: Gunzenhauser N (ed.) Advances in touch. *Johnson & Johnson. Pediatric round table series, Skillman, NJ, pp 11–22*

In the early 1960s, Seymour Levine, Victor Denenberg, and their colleagues published a series of papers describing the effects of postnatal handling on the development of behavioral and endocrine responses to stress. The handling procedure involved removing rat pups from their cages, placing them in small containers, and 15–20 minutes later returning them to their cages and reuniting them with their mothers. This manipulation was peformed once a day for the first 21 days of life. As adults, those rats that had been handled

(H) exhibited less fear in novel environments and a less pronounced increase in the secretion of the adrenal glucocorticoids in response to a variety of stressors than rats that had not been handled (NH). These findings clearly demonstrated that the development of rudimentary adaptive responses to stress could be modified by environmental events. In the studies described here, we have followed on the earlier handling studies, examining the way in which early environmental events alter the development of specific biochemical systems in the brain. We have shown how early handling influences the neurochemical development of certain brain regions that regulate the endocrine response to stress. Neonatal handling increases the efficiency of adaptive endocrine responses to stress, shielding the animal from excessive exposure to the highly catabolic adrenal steroids. In later life, this effect appears to protect the animal from potentially damaging effects of these steroids, ensuring more efficient cognitive functioning.

STROKE

Mok E, Woo CP (2004). The effects of slow-stroke back massage on anxiety and shoulder pain in elderly stroke patients. *Complementary Therapies in Nursing and Midwifery* **10:209–216**

Method: This study explores the effect of slow-stroke back massages on anxiety and shoulder pain in hospitalized elderly patients with stroke. An experimental quantitative design was conducted, comparing the scores for self-reported pain, anxiety, blood pressure, heart rate and pain of two groups of patients before and immediately after, and 3 days after the intervention. The intervention consisted of 10 minutes of slow-stroke back massage (SSBM) for seven consecutive evenings. One hundred and two patients participated in the entire study and were randomly assigned to a massage group or a control group.

Results: The results revealed that the massage intervention significantly reduced the patients' levels of pain perception and anxiety. In addition to the subjective measures, all physiological measures (systolic and diastolic blood pressures and heart rate) changed positively, indicating relaxation. The prolonged effect of SSBM was also evident, as reflected by the maintenance of the psycho-physiological parameters 3 days after the massage. The patients' perceptions of SSBM, determined from a questionnaire, revealed positive support for SSBM for elderly stroke patients. The authors suggest that SSBM is an effective nursing intervention for reducing shoulder pain and anxiety in elderly stroke patients.

SUBSTANCE P

Morhenn VB (2000). Firm stroking of human skin leads to vasodilatation possibly due to the release of substance P. *Journal of Dermatological Science* **22:138–144**

Method: Eight individuals were given a face massage and skin temperature was measured. In seven of eight humans tested, an elevation in the skin's temperature was documented after massaging the cheeks of the face. The elevation of the skin's temperature reached a plateau after about 40 minutes of massaging and was correlated with visible erythema. This effect could be inhibited by repeated pretreatment of the skin with topical capsaicin, a chemical that results in the release of substance P from peripheral nerve endings. Thus, it appears that the temperature elevation induced by stroking of human skin is controlled, at least in part, by release of the neurotransmitter, substance P.

Results: The release of neurotransmitter(s) may be the survival advantage that grooming confers to animals.

SURGERY

Antoniv VR (2002). Effect of neck massage therapy on the soft tissues after thyroid surgery. *Likarska Sprava* **2:93–96**

Our objectives in this study were to establish validated methods of massotherapy of the neck, to determine its action on the neck structures, and to conduct a comparative evaluation of results of the control and study groups after performing massotherapy. It has been found out that in 80 (85%) patients the skin comes to be tinged with healthy pink, the cutaneous-and-muscle tone getting improved, which event makes the skin smooth and elastic following the above massage. Over the first 10 days of the massoprocedures 44 (48%) subjects demonstrated resolution of the edema and swelling, with the thickened skin fold as a roller disappearing by the end of the second month. Dispelling of hypthyrosis phenomena made for reduction of dosages of hormonal preparations. We consider it mandatory that massotherapy of the neck be instituted in all those patients who had undergone operation on the neck and thyroid.

Hattan J, King L, Griffiths P (2002). The impact of foot massage and guided relaxation following cardiac surgery: a randomized controlled trial. *Journal of Advanced Nursing* **37:199–207**

Method: This study investigated the impact of foot massage and guided relaxation on the well-being of patients who had undergone coronary artery bypass graft surgery. Twenty-five subjects were randomly assigned to either a control or one of two intervention groups. Psychological and physical variables were measured immediately before and after the intervention. A discharge questionnaire was also administered.

Results: Increased calm scores occurred for the massage group. There was a clear (non-significant) trend across all psychological variables for both foot massage and, to a lesser extent, guided relaxation to improve psychological well-being. Both interventions were well received by the subjects.

Kim MS, Cho KS, Woo H, et al (2001). Effects of hand massage on anxiety in cataract surgery using local anesthesia. *Journal of Cataract & Refractive Surgery* **27:884–890**

Method: This study comprised 59 patients having cataract surgery. The patients were divided into those having a hand massage 5 minutes before surgery and those not receiving a hand massage. Patients' anxiety levels were measured using the Visual Analog Scale and by assessing systolic blood pressure, diastolic blood pressure, and pulse rate before and after the hand massage and 5 minutes before the end of surgery. Epinephrine, norepinephrine, cortisol, blood sugar levels, neutrophil, and lymphocyte percentages in white blood cells were also measured.

Results: After the hand massage, the psychological anxiety levels, systolic and diastolic blood pressures, and pulse rate were significantly lower than before the massage. The hand massage significantly decreased epinephrine and norepinephrine levels in the experimental group while epinephrine, norepinephrine, and cortisol levels increased in the control group.

TRANSPLANTS

Doering TJ, Fieguth HG, Steuernagel B, et al (1999). External stimuli in the form of vibratory massage after heart or lung transplantation. *American Journal of Physical Medicine Rehabilitation* **78:108–110**

Method: The aim of this pilot study was to examine the influence of manual vibratory massage on the pulmonary function of postoperative patients who were receiving mechanical ventilation, with special interest being focused on pulmonary ventilation and perfusion and cerebral blood flow velocity. Manual vibratory massage was performed postoperatively in the intensive care unit on eight patients: three patients had undergone heart transplantation, three had undergone lung transplantation, and two had undergone coronary artery bypass grafting (mean age 54 years). Changes of respiration parameters and cerebral blood flow velocity (measured by transcranial Doppler sonography) were examined. The vibratory massage was performed with a frequency of 8–10 vibrations/s for 15 minutes, 7.5 minutes on each side of the thorax, starting from the lower costal arch and progressing to the upper thoracic aperture. For 10 minutes before, during, and 10 minutes after the massage, the parameters of peripheral oxygen saturation, central venous pressure, mean arterial pressure, heart rate, lung resistance and compliance, tidal volume, respiration rate, and cerebral blood flow velocity were recorded at 2-minute intervals. Moreover, before and after vibratory massage, arterial blood gases were determined.

Results: In four of the eight patients, it was possible to determine pulmonary arterial pressure, pulmonary capillary wedge pressure, as well as pulmonary vascular resistance. During the vibratory massage, mean tidal volume increased by 30%. Percutaneous oxygen saturation also increased, from 92 to

94%. Central venous pressure decreased by 11%, and pulmonary vessel resistance was reduced by 18%. Pulmonary resistance decreased by the end of the observation period. Thus, vibratory massage seemed to improve pulmonary mechanism and perfusion, thus, reducing ventilation perfusion mismatch and increasing oxygen saturation.

Smith MC, Reeder F, Daniel L, et al (2003). Outcomes of touch therapies during bone marrow transplant. *Alternative Therapies* **9:40–49**

Method: This study investigated the effects of therapeutic touch and massage therapy on the outcomes of engraftment time, complications, and perceived benefits of therapy during bone marrow transplant. Subjects were adult patients on the bone marrow transplant unit of a large urban tertiary care center. Subjects were randomly assigned to one of three treatment groups: therapeutic touch, massage therapy, and a control group called the friendly visit. Subjects (n = 88) were stratified by type of transplant (allogeneic or autologous). Twenty-seven subjects received massage therapy; 31 received therapeutic touch; and 30 received a friendly visit. Nurses with expertise in the two touch therapies administered them. The interventions of massage therapy, therapeutic touch, and friendly visit were administered according to standardized protocols every third day beginning the day chemotherapy began until discharge from the program. Time for engraftment, complications, and patient perceptions of benefits of therapy were the main outcome measures.

Results: A significantly lower score for central nervous system or neurological complications was noted for subjects who received massage therapy compared with the control group; however, no differences were found among the three groups with respect to the other 10 complication categories or in the total mean score for complications. Patients' perception of the benefits of therapy (total score) was significantly higher for those who received massage therapy compared with the friendly visit control group.

VOICE DISORDERS

Ternstrom S, Andersson M, Bergman U (2000). An effect of body massage on voice loudness and phonation frequency in reading. *Logopedics, Phoniatrics, Vocology* **25:146–150**

Method: The effect of massage on voice fundamental frequency and sound pressure level was investigated. Subjects were recorded while reading a 3-minute passage of prose text. Then, a 30-minute session of massage was administered. Sixteen subjects were given the massage, while 15 controls rested, lying in silence for the same amount of time. The subjects were then recorded reading the same passage again.

Results: In the post-massage recordings, subjects had lowered their fundamental frequency and sound pressure level.

YOGA

Khalsa SB (2004). Yoga as a therapeutic intervention: a bibliometric analysis of published research studies. *Indian Journal of Physiology and Pharmacology* **48:269–285**

Review: Although yoga is historically a spiritual discipline, it has also been used clinically as a therapeutic intervention. A bibliometric analysis on the biomedical journal literature involving research on the clinical application of yoga has revealed an increase in publication frequency over the past three decades with a substantial and growing use of randomized controlled trials. Types of medical conditions have included psychopathological (e.g. depression, anxiety), cardiovascular (e.g. hypertension, heart disease), respiratory (e.g. asthma), diabetes and a variety of others. A majority of this research has been conducted by Indian investigators and published in Indian journals, particularly yoga specialty journals, although recent trends indicate increasing contributions from investigators in the U.S. and England. Yoga therapy is a relatively novel and emerging clinical discipline within the broad category of mind–body medicine, whose growth is consistent with the burgeoning popularity of yoga in the West and the increasing worldwide use of alternative medicine.

Telles S, Joshi M, Dash M, et al (2004). An evaluation of the ability to voluntarily reduce the heart rate after a month of yoga practice. *Integrative Physiological and Behavioral Science* **39:119–125**

Method: This study aimed at determining whether novices to yoga would be able to reduce their heart rate voluntarily and whether the magnitude of reduction would be more after 30 days of yoga training. Two groups (yoga and control, n = 12 each) were assessed on Day 1 and on Day 30. During the intervening 30 days, the yoga group received training in yoga techniques while the control group carried on with their routine. At each assessment the baseline heart rate was recorded for 1 minute; this was followed by a 6-minute period during which participants were asked to attempt to voluntarily reduce their heart rate, using any strategy.

Results: Both the baseline heart rate and the lowest heart rate achieved voluntarily during the 6-minute period were significantly lower in the yoga group on Day 30 compared to Day 1 by a group average of 10.7 beats per minute (bpm) and 6.8 bpm, respectively. In contrast, there was no significant change in either the baseline heart rate or the lowest heart rate achieved voluntarily in the control group on Day 30 compared to Day 1.

Index